Bath
SCENTS

ALAN HAYES

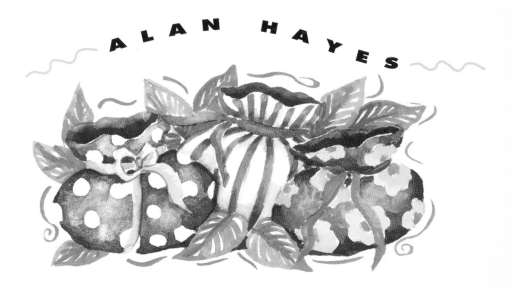

Angus&Robertson

An imprint of HarperCollins*Publishers*

Note: *Neither the author nor the publisher directly or indirectly dispense medical advice or prescribe the use of various herbal remedies. The intent is to provide information that you may wish to explore as a natural alternative. Information about allergic reactions from some herbal products can be found on page 8. If you have any further queries, you should seek the advice of your medical practitioner.*

Angus&Robertson
An imprint of HarperCollins*Publishers*, Australia

First published in Australia in 1994
Reprinted in 1995

Copyright © Alan B. Hayes
Illustrations © Penny Lovelock

HarperCollins*Publishers*
25 Ryde Road, Pymble, Sydney, NSW 2073, Australia
31 View Road, Glenfield, Auckland 10, New Zealand
77-85 Fulham Palace Road, London W6 8JB, United Kingdom
Hazelton Lanes, 55 Avenue Road, Suite 2900, Toronto, Ontario M5R 3L2
and 1995 Markham Road, Scarborough, Ontario M1B 5M8, Canada
10 East 53rd Street, New York NY 10032, USA

National Library of Australia Cataloguing-in-Publication data:

Hayes, Alan B. (Alan Bruce), 1949–
Bath scents.

ISBN 0 207 18230 2.
1. Herbal cosmetics. 2 Essences and essential oils.
3. Herbs – Therapeutic use. 4. Beauty, Personal. I. Title.
646.72

Printed in Hong Kong

10 9 8 7 6 5 4 3 2   95 96 97 98 99

Contents

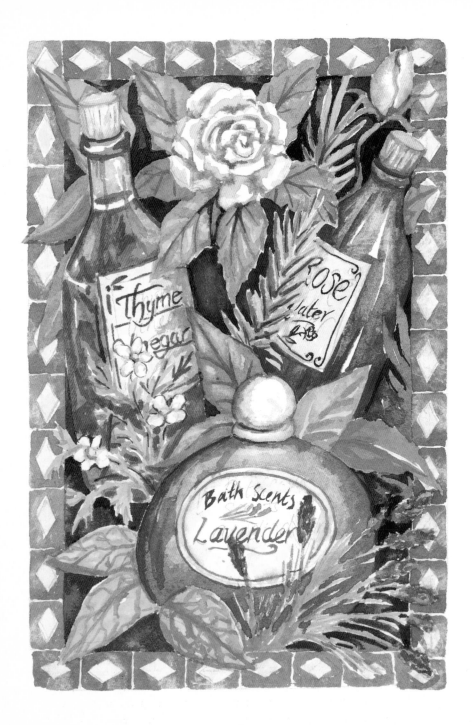

Introduction

Centuries ago, long before bathing was popular as a means of relaxing or of simply coming clean, herbal baths were used as cures for many types of skin problems and other ailments. Today fresh herbs or essential oils can be used in a bath for their toning effect, as a fragrant addition to help you relax, to help ease tired and aching muscles, or to promote healthy, natural sleep.

A bath can be your personal oasis, where the blues simply melt away or you recover from a hard day, and it can be a place to accomplish all those intimate beauty routines you keep promising yourself you'll get around to one of these days. Baths are a wonderful way to restore body energy, soothe the muscles and refresh the skin — in the same way a good night's sleep can.

Year-round body care will result in a smoother and firmer body. Although not everyone can have a wonderful shape, if what you do have is pampered and well cared for, then you will feel attractive. So it is important to use the time you spend in the bath in a profitable and enjoyable way.

As you turn the pages of this book you will discover the delightful ways in which you can become part of the bathing culture. This book takes you from the many uses of herbs and aromatics for all-over skin care, right through to the absolute hedonism of sharing your bath with someone special.

There are indulgent fragrant waters for washing, special scented waters for the bath, and therapeutic blends of oils and herbs to help maintain your skin and keep it soft and supple. And, for something special, there are baths especially for smoothing or moisturising skin. For those in a hurry, there are irresistible aromatic showers, not forgetting a recipe for a real 'get-up-and-go' bath that makes you feel invigorated and alive.

For those of you who might wish to try something different, saunas, jacuzzis and steam rooms are all excellent ways to relax body and soul, as well as being convivial environments for socialising. What better way to throw off the shackles of a hard day's work than to lie back in the soothing and restorative waters of your own hot tub, as you share a glass of your favourite wine under a canopy of stars?

Bath mitts filled with aromatic herbs will add that touch of luxury, filling the air with fragrance while they soften and cleanse your skin. Delightfully fragrant washballs and luxurious aromatic oils will almost make you believe bathing is a sin! And, when you step from your bath or shower, revel in the sheer pleasure of exotic body oils and lotions, or enjoy the astringent bite of a cooling body splash. For a touch of luxury there are body powders that will leave you feeling pampered and alluring.

Natural fragrance in the bathroom gives pure pleasure to your brain, and will help to add a touch of luxury to the time that you spend there.

General Advice About the Recipes

Throughout this book I have endeavoured to keep the various preparations as pure and simple as possible. As a result, you won't end up with a lotion or oil that looks like a commercial product. In most instances the preparations will tend to be plain, with no real colour at all. To add colour is to sacrifice purity for appearance.

Ingredients

If an ingredient or term is unfamiliar to you, look it up in the Glossary at the end of the book. Each term is simply and clearly explained.

Always use distilled water in the recipes, including in the preparation of herb and flower waters. This will prevent any contamination, since tap water contains chemicals and impurities which may interfere with the action of the herbs and other ingredients.

A Word of Advice

For these recipes you will need only basic kitchen equipment, plus other odds and ends you probably also have in your kitchen. However, before you start, you must take these precautions so as not to contaminate or mar the preparations:

* *Do not use aluminium, metal or non-stick pans for boiling or steeping herbs and flowers, or for the preparation of herbal recipes, as they may react chemically with*

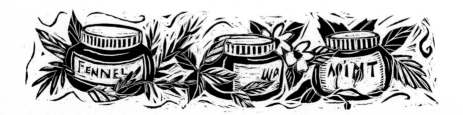

the natural ingredients. Use only stainless steel or enamel pans for boiling, and ceramic or glass pots for steeping.

* All equipment must be kept spotlessly clean, and preferably used only for the preparation of herbal recipes. This safeguards the products from contamination by foodstuffs and other foreign substances. Again, do not use metal or aluminium, and always use a wooden spoon to stir, particularly when heating up ingredients.

* Sterilise all containers and their lids. Use glass jars to store the preparations if you can — they are easier to sterilise.

* Label everything you make with its name and the date on which you made it — don't rely on memory.

* Always use fresh herbs unless dried herbs are specified. When using dried herbs, choose only those with good aroma and colour.

Herb and Flower Waters

The simplest herb water is made by steeping fresh or dried herbs in boiling water, and is known as a 'herbal infusion'. The bark and roots of a plant, however, will not yield their properties by this process; you must use an extraction method called a 'decoction'. The delicate scents of flowers need to be treated differently again, and can be obtained by a variety of methods.

HERBAL INFUSION

Place the selected herbs in a large ceramic bowl and pour boiling water over them. Cover and steep for 12 hours or overnight for a strong infusion, until cool for a weak infusion, or as otherwise directed. Then strain through muslin and add the required amount to the recipe.

The following proportions, unless otherwise directed, should be used:

3 to 4 tablespoons fresh herbs, or
1 to 2 teaspoons dried herbs for every 300 ml
(10 fl oz) of boiling water

Usually, infusions will last only one or two days. However, if they are stored in glass jars in the refrigerator they will last for up to a week. Infusions can be made from one herb or a mixture of herbs, depending on the requirements of a recipe or your particular needs.

Herb Decoction

Put the selected herbs in a stainless steel or enamel pan and add distilled water. Bring to the boil and then simmer gently for 30 minutes. Remove the pan from the heat, cover, and allow the mixture to steep until cold. Strain through muslin and add required amount to recipe.

The following proportions should apply:

3 to 4 tablespoons fresh herbs, or
1 to 2 teaspoons dried herbs for every 300 ml
(10 fl oz) of distilled water

Flower Decoction

This recipe will give you beautifully-scented water from any fragrant flower.

Put 4 tablespoons of fresh petals in an enamel or stainless steel saucepan and cover with 1½ cups (375 ml/12 fl oz) of water. Bring to boiling point, cover and simmer for 30 minutes. Remove from heat, cool, strain through muslin, and squeeze any remaining liquid from the flower petals.

Repeat this process with the same liquid and more fresh petals, depending on the strength and type of flowers used, up to four more times for greater potency. Simply add fresh flowers to the liquid and top up the level.

Flower Water Made in the Oven

Preheat oven to 220°C/435°F. Place 900 g (30 oz) of fresh flower petals or 600 g (20 oz) of dried flowers in a ceramic casserole, cover with distilled water, and place in oven. When the water reaches boiling point, cover with casserole lid and leave in the oven for a further 15 minutes. Remove and allow flower water to cool while covered, then strain through muslin.

Flower Water by Distillation

This method produces a very strong-scented floral water and is especially suitable for making rose water, lavender, marjoram and basil waters.

You will need a large, old-fashioned type of enamel kettle that is boiled on the stove, a length of rubber hose approximately one metre (3 feet) long, a short length of glass tubing (which must fit, tightly, inside the rubber hose), a large shallow basin, and a collection flask or jug.

Put 500 g (16 oz) of fresh, sweet-scented flower petals or herbs in the kettle, half fill with distilled water, replace the lid and seal around edge with plasticine so that no steam can escape. Cut the rubber hose in two so that one length is three times longer than the other, insert the glass tubing between the two lengths of rubber hose and attach the end of the shorter piece of hose to the spout of the kettle.

Place the kettle on the stove over a low heat. Position the basin so that it is higher than the kettle, fill it with ice-cold water and ice cubes, and lay the length of hose through it, letting it hang down into the collection flask. Let the water in the kettle simmer until it has completely evaporated; the glass tube will allow you to observe when no more steam is passing through. Throughout the process, keep the basin topped up with iced water or ice cubes.

In the collection flask you will see two layers: the distilled water and the pure flower essence floating on top of it. Using a blender, whisk this fragrant essence with the distilled water until it is completely emulsified. Shake well before use.

PREPARATION

Before commencing the steam distillation process note that:

Salted flowers and herbs are superior to fresh ones. They reach the full development of their aromatic properties in a shorter time. To salt scented flowers or herbs, spread them evenly on a shallow, flat tray and sprinkle a small quantity of salt over them. Then place the salted material in a glass jar and cover with distilled water. Seal the jar, and allow it to stand overnight. Add the contents of the jar to your kettle 'still', adjusting the distilled water if necessary.

Your final distilled product may have a smoky odour at first. Exposure to the air for a short time — say, 10 to 15 minutes — will remove this. Then keep it in tightly-sealed bottles.

When distilling, ensure that the condensing tube is kept cold. The condensing steam must drip, not run.

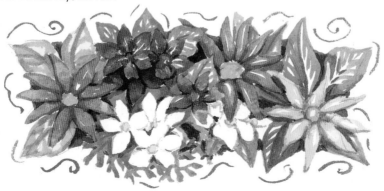

Keeping Herb and Flower Waters

It is important to store herbal waters correctly so they remain as fresh as possible. Being organic, and with no preservatives, they will deteriorate — some more quickly than others. It depends on the plants used. Unless refrigerated, they will usually last only two or three days. There are exceptions, such as lavender, which has good keeping qualities due to its antiseptic properties. Other infusions will keep quite well in a cupboard if blended with an odourless alcohol such as vodka or gin, or if a few drops of benzoin tincture (friar's balsam) are added.

If you add 5 to 10 ml (⅙ to ⅓ oz) of alcohol to every 310 to 500 ml (10 to 16 fl oz) of infusion, or 3 to 4 drops benzoin tincture to every 310 ml (10 fl oz), you can extend the keeping qualities of the mixture. Should you wish to make larger quantities and ensure that the infusion will last indefinitely, add one part alcohol to two parts infusion, stand for 12 hours, then drip the liquid through filter paper.

Unpreserved infusions and shampoo preparations will keep from seven days up to seven months in the refrigerator, providing their containers have been sterilised and are spotlessly clean. But don't leave them and forget about them — check regularly to make sure they haven't gone rancid.

Herb and Flower Vinegars

Vinegars have been used for centuries as bath additives and beauty tonics. They have a far more refreshing scent than floral waters made with alcohol, and they soften both your facial and body skin. Their refreshing quality is due to their acetic acid content, which dissolves the aromatic substances in herbs and flower petals. Aromatic vinegars are best made with a good quality cider vinegar. They can be scented with a wide variety of herbs: rose petals, lavender, rosemary, lemon balm, lemon verbena, basil, hyssop, peppermint, scented geranium leaves and jasmine.

BASIC RECIPE

Half fill a wide-mouthed glass jar with chopped fresh herbs or flower petals and top up with warm vinegar. Seal the jar and leave for 3 to 4 weeks, in a place where it will receive plenty of sunlight. Strain off the vinegar, squeezing all liquid from the herbs. Dilute, if required, according to the recipe directions. If the scent is not strong enough, repeat the process with a fresh batch of herbs or flowers.

For dry herbs or petals, put 3 tablespoons of herbs or 6 tablespoons of petals in a ceramic bowl. Mix 310 ml (10 fl oz) of cider vinegar with the same amount of distilled water, and heat to just below boiling point. Pour the liquid over the herbs, cover tightly with plastic wrap and leave to steep for 12 hours. Strain and bottle.

Herb and floral vinegars will keep indefinitely.

Essential Oils

Essential oils, the life force of all herbs and flowers, are a welcome addition to your bath. Their highly aromatic scents can tantalise, energise or relax, creating just the right atmosphere to suit your mood.

Although pure essential oils are now readily available, you can extract these volatile substances from your own fragrant herbs and flowers, either by simple sun distillation or a process known as 'enfleurage'.

SUN DISTILLATION

Sweet-scented flowers and herbs will yield their aromatic oils by this process.

Place fresh flower petals or herbs in a large, wide-mouthed glass jar and cover with distilled water. Seal the jar with plastic wrap, making sure it is airtight, and leave it where it will receive hot sunlight every day.

When a thin film of oil appears after several days, gently lift it off with cotton wool and squeeze it into a small, amber-coloured glass bottle. Seal the bottle tightly, reseal the distilling jar and continue the process until no more oil appears.

ENFLEURAGE

Pick your fresh herbs or flower petals in the morning after the dew has evaporated, when they are at their most fragrant. Select only perfect specimens, discarding any damaged ones and keeping different types of herbs separated.

Place a layer of petals or herb leaves in the bottom of a small ceramic pot (such as a casserole) — never use glass or metal — and sprinkle a thin layer of coarse salt over them. Repeat the procedure until the vessel is full. Put the lid in place and seal tightly with plasticine or Blu-Tac. Leave undisturbed for a month in a cool, dark cupboard.

After a month, strain the liquid into a glass jar through muslin cloth, squeezing all liquid from the herbs. Seal the jar and leave it, where it will receive plenty of sunlight, for 6 weeks, so that any sediment will settle. You will now have a concentrated fragrant oil.

Decant without disturbing any sediment which may have settled in the bottom of the jar, and strain once more, this time through filter paper.

Keeping Herb and Flower Oils

Essential oils should always be stored in small, amber-coloured, airtight glass bottles, away from heat and light. Never keep mixed oils, and especially those made with carrier oil base, any longer than two months because they begin to oxidise as soon as they are blended.

Allergic Reactions

Due to the prevalence of skin sensitivities and allergic reactions, it is important to test any new substance or ingredient before use. To do this, place a small amount of the substance on the tender skin inside your forearm, then cover it with a bandage for approximately 24 hours. If your skin reddens, burns, itches or blisters, remove the test patch immediately and do not use that ingredient in the recipe.

One of the great advantages of making your own natural products is that if you do have an allergic reaction you know what ingredients you have used, and can, therefore, soon identify the culprit.

Certain vegetable and essential oils may irritate sensitive skin, particularly on the face and around the neck. Those which most commonly cause an allergic reaction are:

ALMOND • BAY LEAF • BERGAMOT • GERANIUM (all types)
• LAVENDER (large doses) • NEROLI • PEPPERMINT
• ROSEMARY (hypersensitive people only) • SAGE • SPEARMINT • THYME

Herbs which may provoke an allergic reaction are:
LIME (linden) BLOSSOMS • LOVAGE • NETTLES • VIOLET LEAVES

Another ingredient which can provoke an allergic reaction is glycerine. If you are in any doubt, consult your doctor.

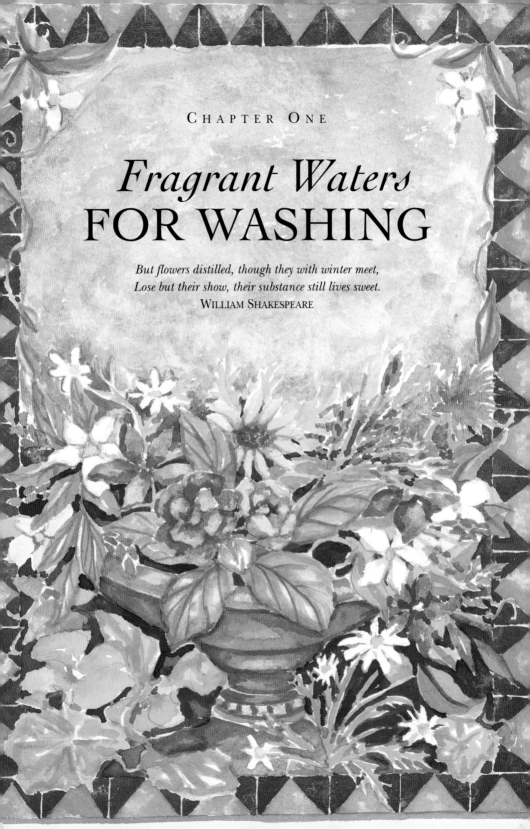

CHAPTER ONE

Fragrant Waters
FOR WASHING

But flowers distilled, though they with winter meet,
Lose but their show, their substance still lives sweet.
WILLIAM SHAKESPEARE

Fragrant Waters for the Complexion

The first recorded use of fragrant water was in 10th century Persia, where it was used for cleansing the face and body. Fragrant waters were also much favoured by English ladies and a basin full of scented washing water was once considered the ultimate luxury in a bedroom or bathroom. Before cutlery as we know it came into use, bowls of scented water were always placed on the tables in manor houses and castles to enable guests to wash their hands between courses.

Scented flowers and herbs may be infused with water, or distilled to make preparations that will cleanse, tone and beautify the skin. Use them without soap to gently cleanse and refresh the complexion last thing at night or first thing in the morning. They will act as tonics for the skin, helping to control overactive sebaceous glands and to close the pores of the skin, thus firming the skin and redressing its pH balance at the same time.

Herbs and Their Properties

Sweet-scented washing waters are easy to make at home by either distillation, infusion or decoction, or through the simple addition of aromatic oils. Herbs and flowers you can try are:

CHAMOMILE — *Slightly antiseptic and particularly beneficial to people with oily skin, especially when blended with equal amounts of rosemary. Regular bathing helps to reduce and smooth out wrinkles and tone up relaxed muscles.*

COMFREY
WITCH HAZEL — *Helps smooth out wrinkles and will act as a tonic for the skin.*

ELDER FLOWER — *Acts as a mild astringent, and is particularly good to use after cleansing the skin.*

LEMON BALM — *Helps smooth out wrinkles.*

LIME FLOWER — *Helps smooth out wrinkles.*

NETTLE — *Has good cleansing and toning qualities for the skin, leaving it with a refreshing tingle.*

ROSEMARY — *Acts as a tonic to tighten up sagging skin.*

ROSE PETALS	*Soothe and soften the skin and are especially good after exposure to strong winds or sun. Rose Petal water also makes a refreshing bath for the eyes.*
SAGE	*Is invigorating and cleansing.*
THYME	*Acts as an astringent and helps to clear spots and acne.*
WOODRUFF	*Freshens the complexion and soothes the skin after exposure to sun or wind.*
YARROW	*Good for oily and greasy skin. Acts as a light astringent.*

Fresh or Dried Herbs

Fresh and dried herbs are equally effective in making beautifully scented waters. Use any of the methods described in the Introduction, choosing only perfect specimens with good colour and aroma.

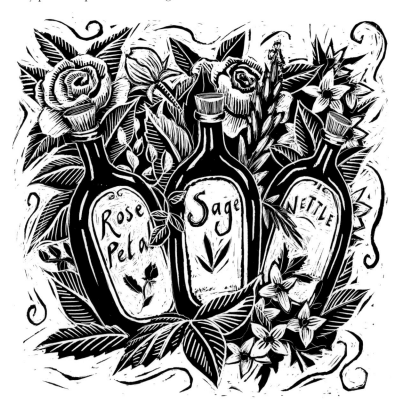

SWEET SCENTED WATER

My wife uses this water as a final rinse after shampooing her hair, and quite often for washing her face, too. It will work best as a facial tonic if you do as she does, and use a small natural sponge to pat on the liquid. And, if you're feeling really indulgent, add a cup or two to your bath water.

Fill a large, wide-mouthed glass jar with fresh, strongly-scented rose petals and a handful of lavender buds. Add 1 teaspoon of whole cloves, 1 crushed whole nutmeg and a pinch of mace. Top up the jar with distilled water. Seal the jar so that it is airtight, and leave it in a sunny spot for 3 days. Shake the contents every day, then process in the 'kettle still' as described on pages 4–5. If necessary, adjust the quantity of distilled water before commencing distillation.

Fragrant Waters from Aromatic Oils

Adding an essential oil to soft water is the easiest way to make a sweet-scented washing water. Add 6 drops of your chosen oil to every 625 ml (20 fl oz) of water. Shake the mixture well and leave it for 12 hours before using. Shake well again before use.

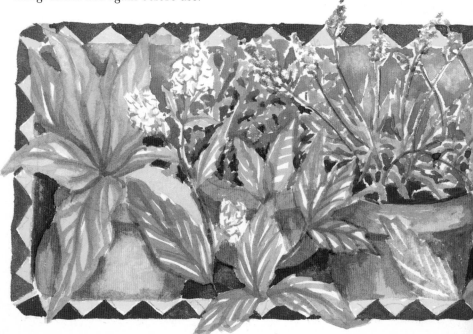

If you dissolve the essential oil in a small quantity of perfumer's alcohol or vodka before adding it to the distilled water, it will be completely emulsified in the liquid and will not require shaking before use. Use 5 ml (⅙ fl oz/ 1 teaspoon) of alcohol to every 2.5 litres (4¼ pints) of water or part thereof.

Scents to Use

Choosing aromatic oils for washing waters is purely a matter of personal taste. Be sure to choose only pure oils, not synthetic ones or those diluted with a base oil or alcohol.

The advantage of using essential oils is that you can quickly and easily make up several different scented waters to use according to your mood or the time of day. Rose or lavender alone, or combined, are suitable at any time. Essential oil of rose will soften the skin and also has a relaxing and calming effect, while lavender both relaxes and exerts natural disinfectant qualities. Mixed with peppermint or rosemary, lavender acts as an early morning refresher. Rosemary mixed with basil or marjoram has a clean fresh scent, while other herbs, such as violet or rosewood, can be enjoyed for their delightful and delicate perfumes.

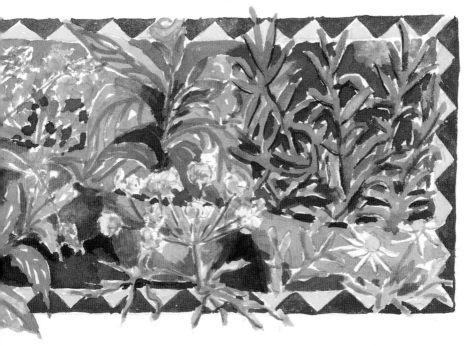

Scented Waters for the Bath

Herb and floral waters can also be added to your bath — and lying back in an aromatic bath is surely one of life's greatest pleasures! Depending on which herbs you use, a bath can relax and calm, or revive and invigorate. It can ease tired, aching limbs and sore muscles, or stimulate the circulation.

Making up a fresh infusion each time you have a bath is not very practical, so it is best to ensure your scented waters are long lasting. This can be done by adding either vodka or cider vinegar to the water. Vinegar is more astringent and therefore ideal for people who have oily skin.

For every 600 ml (20 fl oz) of liquid you will need to use 3 tablespoons of dried herbs or 6 tablespoons of dried flower petals. Put the herbs in an enamel pan, add 300 ml (10 fl oz) each of distilled water and cider vinegar and heat to just below boiling point; cover and simmer for 10 minutes. Remove mixture from heat and allow to cool, then seal the top of the pan with plastic wrap and steep for 12 hours. Strain mixture through fine muslin, squeezing the herbs to extract as much liquid as possible. Store in an attractive bottle with a ground glass stopper.

Alternatively, substitute distilled water for the cider vinegar and follow the same procedure, adding 85 ml (3 fl oz) of vodka to every 625 ml (20 fl oz) of liquid or part thereof.

Add 155 ml (5 fl oz) of the scented water to your bath while the taps are running.

Herbs to Use

You can use herbs singly or in combination, according to preference and need. Choose from: rosemary, lavender, lemon balm, hyssop, chamomile, elder flowers, honeysuckle, lovage, lime flowers, peppermint, rose petals or any of the sweet-scented geranium leaves.

LAVENDER BATH WATER

Add this fragrant water to your bath to relieve sore muscles and prevent skin dryness.

Put 2 generous handfuls of dried lavender buds in a ceramic bowl. Mix together 500 ml (16 fl oz) each of distilled water and cider vinegar in a non-metallic saucepan and bring to just below boiling point. Pour the liquid over the herbs, seal the bowl with plastic wrap and allow to steep for

12 hours. Strain mixture through fine muslin, squeezing all liquid from the herbs; bottle for future use.

Add 1 cup (250 ml/8 fl oz) of lavender water to your bath while the taps are running.

BATH WATER FOR RELAXATION

Add this scented water to an evening bath when you need to relax after a hard day. It will calm and soothe you, and help promote a good night's sleep.

Put 1 tablespoon each of dried lavender, rose and chamomile in a ceramic bowl, add 500 ml (16 fl oz) of boiling water, cover and steep for 10 minutes. Strain through muslin and add the liquid to a warm bath.

DID YOU KNOW . . . ?

That sweet washing waters were once a luxury for only the rich to enjoy? However, after the Great Plague that affected Europe during the 17th century, they became popular among all classes when it was realised that cleanliness was not only 'next to godliness' but also played an important role in keeping disease away.

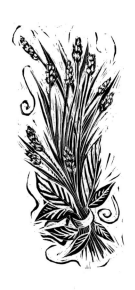

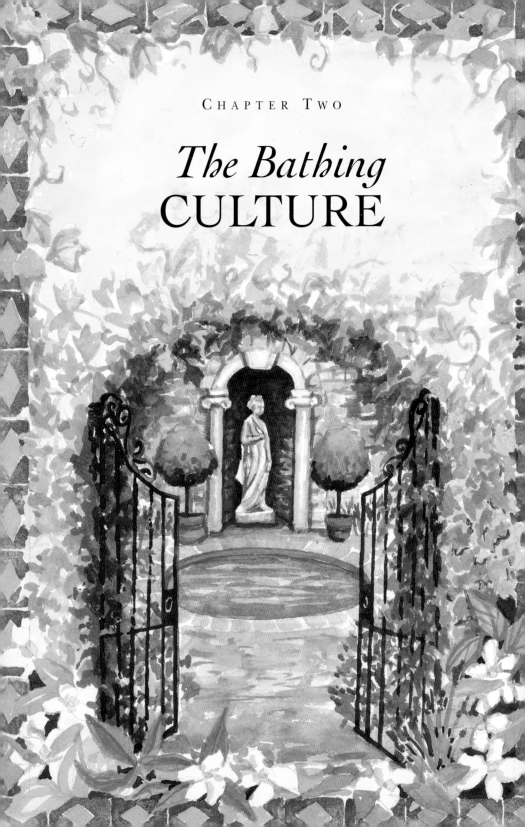

CHAPTER TWO

The Bathing CULTURE

Herbal Baths

Many of us enjoy relaxing in a luxurious bath at the end of a long day, or even having a quick, refreshing bath before a day's work. Whatever your bathing habits are, it is important to avoid extremes of temperature. Water that is too hot or too cold can be a shock to the system, and may cause overstimulation of the sebaceous glands or damage delicate blood vessels. Have the water comfortably warm, so that a splash with tepid water should be enough to close the pores.

Herbs added to the bath water provide a delightful fragrance, and also cleanse, beautify and tone your skin, or relax or invigorate your whole body while you soak. Although fresh herbs may look pretty scattered in your bathwater, there is a problem when you have to remove them. Allowing them to simply disappear down the plughole could eventually result in a blocked drain. Instead, add your herbs in the form of a sweet-scented water (see Chapter One), or in a bath bag. You can use either fresh or dried herbs.

To make a bath bag, take a 20 cm (8 in) square of muslin, place the herbs in the centre and draw up the sides, securing the bag with a piece of ribbon. For maximum effect, hang the bag from the tap so that the hot water gushes through it. Rub the bag briskly over your body like a sponge, and then lie back and relax in the fragrant water.

Mint, rosemary and lavender will help revitalise the skin and energise the body by stimulating the circulation. Jasmine, chamomile and elder flowers will soothe, soften and calm the skin, while a mixture of pine needles and peppermint will leave you feeling refreshed and invigorated.

Other Additives

OILS: *There is a whole range of exotic, mysterious or romantic scented oils that will make your bath something special, whether you are alone or sharing the experience. Their many properties and benefits are detailed in Chapter Four.*

VINEGARS: *Aromatic vinegars will leave your skin feeling wonderfully soft. Chapter Five details their many uses.*

SALT: *A generous handful of sea salt is particularly beneficial if you have any broken or sore skin or scars that need to be healed.*

Herbs for Your Individual Needs

ANGELICA	*Invigorating and rejuvenating.*
BAY LEAVES	*Aromatic; comforts aching limbs.*
BLACKBERRY LEAVES	*Very invigorating.*
BORAGE, SAGE AND TANSY	*Enlivening.*
CHAMOMILE	*Very soothing and relaxing; calms the nerves.*
COMFREY	*Invigorating, rejuvenating and cleansing.*
ELDER FLOWERS	*Healing and stimulating.*
EUCALYPTUS LEAVES	*Aromatic.*
HONEYSUCKLE	*Aromatic; softens the skin.*
HYSSOP	*Relieves stiffness.*
JUNIPER	*Invigorating.*
LAVENDER	*Aromatic with a clean, refreshing scent; natural disinfectant; softens the skin.*
LEMON BALM	*Very relaxing.*
LIME FLOWERS	*Very calming.*
LOVAGE	*Invigorating, rejuvenating, relaxing and a mild natural deodorant.*
MARJORAM	*Aromatic.*
NETTLE LEAVES	*Invigorating and rejuvenating.*
PENNYROYAL	*Refreshing scent; comforts the nerves.*
PEPPERMINT	*Extra invigorating.*
PINE NEEDLES	*Extra invigorating, with a clean, fresh scent.*
PLANTAIN LEAVES	*Healing; use for skin ailments.*
ROSE PETALS	*Will make the water fragrant and sweet while also softening the skin.*

ROSEMARY	*Stimulates the circulation, softens the skin, relieves stiff joints and relaxes aching muscles.*
SAGE	*Aromatic and cleansing.*
SCENTED GERANIUM LEAVES	*There are many varieties of this beautifully scented herb. Their different fragrances will add a touch of the exotic to your bath, with wonderful smells of lemon, coconut, rose, spice, lime, mint and musk, to name but a few.*
THYME	*Delightful aromatic scent.*
VALERIAN	*Very soothing, relaxing and cleansing; has a bitter scent.*
VIOLETS	*Aromatic.*
YARROW	*Cleansing and soothing.*

Preparations for Special Purposes

The following herbal bath suggestions may all be added to a bath in a bath bag or as a strong infusion (see page 3). Vary the combinations to suit your own requirements.

A REFRESHING BATH • *Spearmint, lavender, lemon verbena, salad burnet.*

TO EASE TIRED AND ACHING MUSCLES • *Rosemary, bay leaf, honeysuckle, hyssop, angelica, lovage, chamomile.*

TO INVIGORATE AND REJUVENATE • *Rosemary, lovage, lavender, nettle, valerian, peppermint, comfrey.*

TO RELAX, SOOTHE, CALM AND PROMOTE SLEEP • *Chamomile, lovage, lime flowers, pennyroyal, rosemary, yarrow.*

For a relaxing bath, take some finely ground oatmeal and cook it until it is soft, then transfer the mixture to a muslin bag. Hang the bag in the bath water so the liquid can work its soothing magic.

TO COMFORT FRAZZLED NERVES • *Pennyroyal, rosemary, bay leaf, chamomile, lime flowers, valerian.*

TO SOOTHE SORE SKIN • *Comfrey, marigold (calendula), woodruff, violets, lady's mantle, marshmallow, chamomile, elder flowers.*

SWEET BATH WATER • *Chamomile, rosemary, bay leaf, sage.*

JUDITH'S SWEET BATH WATER

These are the herbs my wife mixes together in a strong infusion whenever she feels like luxuriating in a warm bath. This combination will relax body and soul, ease tired and aching limbs and leave your skin smelling wonderfully fragrant.

Combine equal quantities of rose petals, citrus peel, chamomile, orange blossoms, jasmine, bay leaf, rosemary, lavender and peppermint.

Smoothing Baths

Bath time is the ideal time to give some extra attention to rough skin on knees, elbows and heels. Take care of those dead skin cells and get the circulation moving with a pumice stone, loofah or loofah mitt.

If skin cleansing and smoothing is needed, try an oatmeal bath bag. Simply put 2 tablespoons of medium ground oatmeal and 2 tablespoons of dried herbs of your choice in the centre of a 20 cm (8 in) square of muslin, draw up the sides and secure the bag with a piece of ribbon. Then rub any dry skin areas with the moistened bag while relaxing in your bath.

Oatmeal is a well-known skin softener, and you will actually feel the impurities and rough skin float away when you use this treatment.

Loofahs

A loofah (*Luffa aegyptiaca*), or vegetable sponge, is the dry, fibrous part of a gourd. It is very effective for cleaning the whole body. Use a loofah in the bath or shower for sloughing off dead skin cells and improving circulation. You can buy loofahs whole or cut up into smaller pads, or as mitts, with a towelling surface on one side and the fibre surface on the other. Once wet, loofahs swell up and can be used to thoroughly cleanse areas which are susceptible to spots, such as the back and chest.

Growing your own loofahs is simple and inexpensive. They are a quick-growing annual, somewhat like a zucchini. They are easiest to manage if given something to climb on, such as a fence or trellis.

The fruit is ready to harvest for sponge-making when the stalk shrivels. Cut off the stem end, remove the seeds and hang it in a sheltered spot, such as a verandah, so that it will dry naturally in the sun. The fruit will turn yellow and wither and the skin will flake off, leaving the sponge-like fibres. Soak the sponge in clean water overnight, wash it thoroughly in hot, soapy water and rinse it clean. Dry it in the sun and it is ready to use.

Keep your loofah in good condition by washing it occasionally in warm water, to which has been added a little bicarbonate of soda. Rinse it thoroughly in clean, warm water.

LOOFAH BATH TREATS

To relax tired, aching muscles and joints, dissolve 435 g (14 oz) of Epsom salts in a warm bath then add 2 drops each of rosemary oil, bay leaf oil and rose oil, and 4 drops of hyssop oil. Lightly massage your body all over with a loofah or loofah mitt, then lie back and relax in the scented water.

For a more invigorating bath, substitute sea salt for the Epsom salts then add 6 drops of lavender oil and 2 drops each of rosewood oil and tangerine oil.

Exfoliation — the sloughing off of dead skin cells — cleans and 'polishes' the skin, helps to stimulate the circulation and creates a feeling of wellbeing.

Dry Bathing

Dry bathing consists of brushing all parts of the body below the neck with a loofah, with the exception of the delicate breast area in women. Go very gently and lightly on the paler, softer areas of the stomach and inside areas of the arms and legs. Over the rest of the body, use a gentle yet firm pressure, and brush in a rhythmic circular motion.

Each morning on rising, brush the skin for 5 to 10 minutes to stimulate the circulation and rid the body of accumulated dead cells and toxins. Finish off by gently applying a coating of almond or apricot kernel oil all over your body. Leave for 10 minutes, then towel off the excess with a vigorous rub.

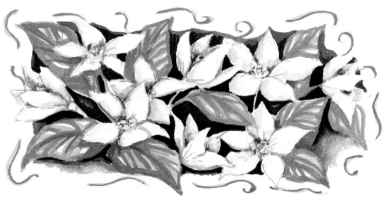

Moisturising Baths

Skin suffers from the harshness of winter, the cold winds leaving it dry and rough. All those clothes that we pile on to keep warm do nothing for our skin either; once they are peeled off, a grey pallor, complete with rough, cracked areas, is often revealed.

The simplest way to moisturise the body while bathing is to add a few drops of almond oil to the water. Your skin will soon be looking and feeling supple again.

You can moisturise and nourish your skin at the same time by adding a teaspoon of the following blend of oils to your bath:

10 ml (⅓ fl oz) avocado oil
10 ml (⅓ fl oz) apricot kernel oil
30 ml (1 fl oz) almond oil
50 drops rose or lavender oil

Thoroughly mix all the oils and store in an amber-coloured, airtight glass bottle. Keep away from direct heat and use within 2 months. Add 1 teaspoon of the mixture to your bath.

Soda Baths

Soda baths are marvellous for soothing itching skin, and for relieving vaginitis, and for children who are allergic to commercial bubble baths. They can be perfumed with aromatic oils or used in combination with fragrant and therapeutic herbs.

To prepare a soda bath, add ½ cup (125 g/4 oz) of bicarbonate of soda to the bath water, swish it around until it dissolves, then lie back and relax. Alternatively (you need to prepare this the day before your bath!), put the bicarbonate of soda in a glass jar, dip the tip of a cotton bud in your favourite aromatic oil and then place it in the soda, making a figure of eight so as to thoroughly distribute the oil. Seal the jar and let it stand for 12 hours. The soda will take on the aroma and perfume your bath (see Chapter Three).

Herbs can also be added to bath water by way of an infusion (to prepare, see Chapter One). For itchy skin, choose a cooling herb such as peppermint. Marshmallow and aloe vera are both excellent for skin irritations and vaginitis.

Cosmetic Baths

This is an ideal bath to cleanse and soften the skin.

25 g (1 oz) barley
100 g (3½ oz) bran
1 handful borage leaves
1 litre (32 fl oz) distilled water

Put all the ingredients in an enamel or stainless steel pan, bring to the boil, cover, and simmer for 10 to 15 minutes. Cool the mixture and then strain it through fine muslin, squeezing all liquid from the ingredients. Add the liquid to the bath while the taps are running. Adding a few drops of your favourite aromatic oil as well will leave your skin smelling fragrant.

Vinegar Baths

This special addition to your favourite herbal bath will help combat dryness of the skin by restoring its acid balance.

10 ml (⅓ fl oz) herbal vinegar
90 ml (3 fl oz) distilled water

Prepare the vinegar using herbs of your choice (see Chapter Five). Combine the vinegar with the distilled water, pour into a suitable bottle and cap securely; shake until well blended.

Brush the skin with the vinegar, using a loofah as you would for dry bathing. This will help loosen dead skin cells and improve circulation. Then rinse off any residue in a warm bath.

Therapeutic Baths

Essential oils added to your bath water release their special properties to penetrate your skin, as well as exerting their therapeutic value through the vapour you inhale. For maximum effect, close all windows and the bathroom door.

If you are ill, nauseated or running a fever, it is not advisable to take a full bath; instead, sponge off underarms and genitals. However, a therapeutic bath can do wonders in speeding up recovery if you are suffering from a cold, a stuffed-up nose, aching muscles and joints, or when you feel generally tired and run-down.

There are detailed instructions on how to prepare aromatic bath oils in Chapter Four. The simplest and quickest method is to dilute 30 drops of your favourite essential oil with 2 tablespoons of almond oil, then add about 10 drops of the blended oil to your bath while the taps are running. Try the following combinations for different therapeutic purposes:

CALMING AND SOOTHING
2 drops rosemary oil
2 drops bay leaf oil
4 drops lime flower oil
2 drops pennyroyal oil

RELAXING EVENING BATH
2 drops chamomile oil
2 drops rose oil
6 drops lavender oil

TO PROMOTE SLEEP
6 drops chamomile oil
2 drops lovage oil
2 drops lime flower oil

TO EASE TIRED AND ACHING MUSCLES
2 drops rosemary oil
2 drops bay leaf oil
2 drops rose oil
4 drops hyssop oil

TO RELIEVE STIFFNESS FROM SPORT
5 drops hyssop oil
2 drops bay leaf oil
3 drops rosemary oil

TO INVIGORATE AND REJUVENATE
6 drops lavender oil
2 drops rosewood or lovage oil
2 drops tangerine oil

THERAPEUTIC BLEND FOR COLDS
6 drops pine oil
6 drops eucalyptus oil
6 drops cypress oil

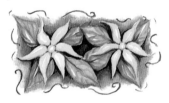

Run bath water as hot as you can stand it; when the bath is almost full, add the pure essential oils.

Sit with your knees up and your head between them so that you can fully inhale the restorative vapours. As the water cools, slosh it all over your body. Then get out of the bath and dry yourself vigorously with a warm towel. Wrap yourself in another warm towel for a few minutes.

To finish, rub your entire body with the following oil blend:

125 ml (4 fl oz) almond oil
2 drops eucalyptus oil
3 drops lavender oil
2 drops thyme oil

Aromatic Showers

Even if your daily schedule doesn't always allow for a relaxing bath, you can still enjoy the benefits of fragrant oils with an aromatic shower.

To start, rub your entire body with a little bath oil containing stimulating or relaxing essences — choose one of the Therapeutic Bath blends on page 24— and dilute it half-and-half with water. Plug the shower drain hole and, while showering, sprinkle in more of the same aromatic oil as the water collects. Your feet will benefit from the fragrant soak, while the ascending aroma will bring pure pleasure to your senses.

Shower Beauty Scrubs

This face scrub is ideal when you are in a hurry, since you need only a few minutes to massage it into the skin.

OATMEAL FACE SCRUB
4 tablespoons fuller's earth
2 tablespoons oatmeal
4 tablespoons mixture of finely ground
herbs — chamomile, rosemary and elder flowers
12 drops lemon juice
aloe vera juice
almond oil
wheatgerm oil
natural yoghurt
1½ tablespoons brewer's yeast

Mix all ingredients, adding sufficient yoghurt, seed oils and aloe vera juice to form a thick paste. Apply to your face and neck, avoiding the area around the eyes and any broken skin. Massage lightly into your skin for 5 minutes and then remove by rinsing thoroughly.

Tone and firm your skin with a mild astringent to close the pores, then smooth in a moisturiser to keep your skin supple and help prevent wrinkles.

CHAMOMILE OATMEAL SCRUB

This scrub will thoroughly cleanse oily skin and leave it glowing. Gently massage the scrub into your arms, legs, face and other parts of your body just before taking a bath or shower. It will help exfoliate and soften the skin, making it more receptive to a body lotion.

This scrub is gentle and mild, and is especially suitable for facial skin and for under the chin and the neck area.

⅔ cup (100 g/3½ oz) oatmeal
1 tablespoon chamomile infusion
3 tablespoons warm milk

Prepare the infusion as directed in the Introduction, page 3, using 1 tablespoon of dried herb to 310 ml (10 fl oz) of boiling water.

Grind the oatmeal to a fine powder then mix it with 1 tablespoon of the infusion and the warm milk to form a paste. Adjust the amounts of milk and oatmeal if necessary. After application, rinse off in bath or shower.

Any leftover chamomile infusion can be added to your bath water.

ALL OVER BODY SCRUB

Use this body scrub in the shower once a week to stimulate the circulation and to slough off dead skin cells.

1 handful cooking salt
almond oil

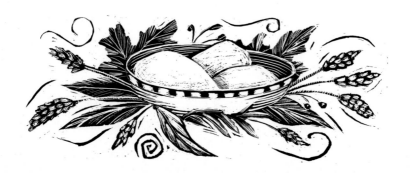

Put the salt in a ceramic bowl and add just enough almond oil to form a paste, mixing thoroughly.

In the shower, massage the paste all over your body, then wash off with lukewarm water. The salt will cleanse the skin and the almond oil has a moisturising effect. Your skin will feel soft and dewy for days.

LEMON AND SALT SCRUB

Use this body scrub before showering to whisk away the uppermost skin cells, then rinse off. It will make your skin more receptive to any of the After Bath Oils described in Chapter Seven.

1 ripe avocado
50 g (2 oz) fine sea salt
3 drops lemon oil

Mash up the avocado in a mixing bowl, then add the salt and lemon oil, mixing thoroughly to form a paste. Rub handfuls of the mixture vigorously over your body, then rinse off in the shower. Finish with a body lotion.

Therapeutic Foot Baths

Your feet communicate with the rest of your body, so a foot massage, combined with a therapeutic footbath, will revive your entire system as well as your tired and swollen feet.

Before soaking your feet, give each one a preliminary massage. Do this while sitting comfortably: place one foot over your knee and press, rub and pull each toe, then knead the sole with your knuckles. Next, place the fingers of both hands on the sole, and the thumbs, pointing toward the toes, on top of the foot. Stroke down from the ankles to the toes.

Now put your feet in the basin and soak them for 15 minutes. Remove one foot at a time, drying each carefully and then rubbing gently with the following massage oil:

CALENDULA FOOT OIL

90 ml (3 fl oz) almond oil
5 ml (⅙ fl oz) avocado oil
2 ml (1/12 fl oz) calendula (marigold) oil

Combine the oils in an airtight amber-coloured glass bottle and shake vigorously until the mixture is completely emulsified.

SOOTHING FOOT BATH

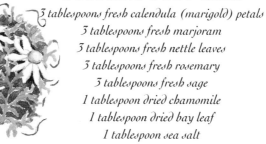

3 tablespoons fresh calendula (marigold) petals
3 tablespoons fresh marjoram
3 tablespoons fresh nettle leaves
3 tablespoons fresh rosemary
3 tablespoons fresh sage
1 tablespoon dried chamomile
1 tablespoon dried bay leaf
1 tablespoon sea salt

Place all the ingredients in a bowl which will be large enough for your feet, then pour the boiling water over them. Cover the bowl and allow the mixture to steep for 30 minutes, then strain it and discard the herbs. Bring herbal liquid to the boil in a stainless steel or enamel pan; pour it back into the bowl, stir in the sea salt until dissolved, and leave to cool slightly before soaking your feet.

After 10 minutes, revive your feet with a quick dip into a basin of cold water, then put them back in the foot bath again. Continue doing this as long as the hot water stays hot, then finish off with a cold dip.

AROMATIC FOOT BATH

4 tablespoons fresh pennyroyal
4 tablespoons fresh sage
4 tablespoons fresh rosemary
4 tablespoons fresh juniper berries
3 tablespoons fresh calendula (marigold) petals
3 tablespoons fresh angelica
1 tablespoon sea salt

Prepare and use as for *Soothing Foot Bath.*

COMFORTING FOOT BATH

1 handful of each of the following fresh herbs:
rosemary
lavender
sage
scented geranium leaves of your choice (optional)
dried chamomile
1 tablespoon washing soda crystals

Prepare as for *Aromatic* and *Soothing Foot Baths,* adding the washing soda after the herbs have been infused and strained and the liquid reheated.

A tablespoon of sea salt is comforting to tired, sore feet, while a pinch or two of mustard powder is invigorating, especially if you have come in with cold, wet feet.

Using Dried Herbs

All the fresh herbs in these foot bath recipes can be replaced with dried herbs. Add them in the following quantities:

LEAVES AND PETALS
1 tablespoon of dried herb for 3 to 4 tablespoons of fresh herb.
BERRIES
1 teaspoon of dried berries to 4 tablespoons of fresh berries.

REVIVING COLD AND TIRED FEET

My grandmother was a great believer in this old-fashioned mustard bath recipe for reviving cold and tired feet.

Blend 3 teaspoons of mustard powder with sufficient water to form a paste. Add to a bowl of hot water and soak your feet for 15 minutes. Finish with a quick dip in a basin of cold water, then gently dry and massage your feet with *Calendula Foot Oil* (see page 27).

HEALING FOOT BATH

An ideal foot bath for fungal conditions such as tinea, an infection which thrives when the skin's acid to alkaline balance has tilted too far in the alkaline direction.

30 g (1 oz) dried soapwort root
3 tablespoons dried chamomile
1 litre (32 fl oz) water
2 litres (64 fl oz) boiling water

Bring the soapwort to the boil in 1 litre (32 fl oz) of water in an enamel or stainless steel pan. Cover and simmer for 25 minutes. Remove mixture from heat, and place in a foot basin, then add the chamomile and 2 litres (64 fl oz) of boiling water. Cover and steep for 30 minutes, then strain. Reheat and pour back into the foot basin. Soak your feet for 15 minutes.

Rinse your feet in a basin of cold water to which has been added 2 tablespoons of cider vinegar. Dry your feet thoroughly with a towel which must be kept for your use only, then boil the towel to reduce the risk of infection.

Dust between your toes with powdered arrowroot when they are thoroughly dried.

SKIN TREATMENT FOOT BATH

Use this for other skin problems with your feet, such as dry or cracked skin or other fungal infections. It will help to restore the acid balance of the skin.

30 g (1 oz) agrimony
30 g (1 oz) onion, finely chopped
30 g (1 oz) sage
30 g (1 oz) red clover blossoms
3 litres (4 ¾ pints) water
2 tablespoons cider vinegar

Combine herbs and water in an enamel or stainless steel pan and simmer for 20 minutes. Strain the mixture through muslin, squeezing all liquid from the herbs, and set the herb pulp and the liquid aside to cool. When the liquid has cooled, stir in the cider vinegar and pour into a suitable basin. Soak your feet for 15 minutes. Remove your feet and rest them on a towel, then pack the herb pulp between your toes, leaving it there for 20 minutes. Rinse your feet in a basin of clean water to which has been added 2 tablespoons of cider vinegar. Dry them thoroughly.

Using Essential Oils

Find a basin which is large enough to hold your feet comfortably. Pour in sufficient warm water to cover them up to your ankles. Depending on how you feel, or your particular need, add the appropriate oils and soak your feet for 20 minutes.

For the maximum beneficial effect, massage your feet before soaking, and finish with the *Calendula Foot Oil*.

HEALING FOOT BATH

Use this therapeutic bath for feet that are battered and bruised, or if you suffer from corns, bunions or inflamed joints. It will help to both heal and strengthen the feet.

1 cup (20 g/8 oz) bicarbonate of soda
5 drops thyme oil

Dissolve the bicarbonate of soda in a basin of warm water, add the thyme oil, then soak your feet for 20 minutes. Finish by dipping your feet briefly into a basin of cold water to refresh them.

SPA FOOT BATH

3 tablespoons Epsom salts
1 tablespoon sea salt
3 drops peppermint oil
1 drop rosemary oil

Add both the salts to a basin of hot water, stirring until they are dissolved. Then add the essential oils, swishing the water to mix them in well. Soak your feet for 10 minutes.

TIRED FEET

Soaking your feet in this blend will soon soothe away tiredness. It is ideal for those who are on their feet all day.

1 tablespoon bicarbonate of soda
3 drops rosemary oil

Dissolve the bicarbonate of soda in a basin of warm water and add the essential oil. Soak your feet for 20 minutes. Finish by giving them a quick dip in a basin of cold water.

SWOLLEN FEET

Three drops of lavender oil in a basin of iced water will help ease swollen and sore feet.

Following is a list of other oils to use. Add 3 to 6 drops of your selected oil (singly or in combination) to a basin of warm water and soak your feet for 20 minutes.

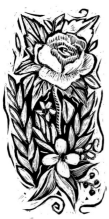

BAY LEAF — *Comforts aching and tired feet.*

CALENDULA — *Heals and rejuvenates.*

HYSSOP — *Relieves stiffness, especially that due to sport.*

JASMINE — *Soothes and relaxes.*

JUNIPER — *Refreshes, stimulates and invigorates.*

LEMONGRASS — *Refreshes, revives and uplifts; heals skin complaints.*

LOVAGE — *Relaxes; natural deodorant properties.*

ROSE — *Relaxes; softens the skin.*

Put Your Best Foot Forward

It is not always possible to sit down and soak your feet in a soothing or healing foot bath. The following tips will help keep your feet in good condition:

* *Rub rosemary oil or diluted apple cider vinegar into your feet, massaging for about 5 minutes before you take a bath.*

* *For dry skin, wash your feet with a mixture of 1 tablespoon of bran and 3 tablespoons of strong chamomile infusion (about 3 level tablespoons of dried chamomile to 310 ml [10 fl oz] of boiling water). Rinse, wipe dry, then moisturise.*

* *To soften extra-hard skin on the soles of the feet or the backs of the heels, massage with equal quantities of olive oil and apple cider vinegar.*

* *Rub the soles of aching feet with apple cider vinegar or lemon juice.*

* *Dust corn flour over blisters to soothe them, and help the healing process.*

* *Rub wheatgerm oil into cracked toenails each night.*

* *Prevent foot odour and excessive perspiration by ensuring that you have sufficient silica in your diet. Include barley, kelp, garlic, onion, parsley, lettuce, alfalfa and strawberries — all are good sources of this mineral.*

SOOTHING FOOT BALM
5 ml (⅙ fl oz) malt vinegar
200 g (6½ fl oz) natural yoghurt

Stir the vinegar into the yoghurt and rub the mixture over your feet and between your toes, massaging in well. Leave for 5 minutes, then rinse off with lukewarm water.

Caring for Hands

Hand Bath

Hands can suffer badly from the daily chores they are expected to perform, and the skin can easily split or crack, becoming dry and leathery. Soaking your hands for 10 minutes each day in a bowl of warm water to which healing or therapeutic oils have been added will keep them in tiptop condition.

Add 2 to 4 drops of any of the following oils to a basin of warm water:

DRY HANDS	NEGLECTED HANDS
rose	*rose*
geranium	*lemon*
carrot	*geranium*

After soaking your hands in the scented hand bath, dry them thoroughly and apply the following hand lotion:

LEMON HAND LOTION
equal quantities of:
lemon juice
glycerine
rose-water

Mix all ingredients together thoroughly and store in an airtight amber-coloured glass bottle. Massage generously into hands and wrists.

This lotion moisturises and softens the hands and, as a bonus, also strengthens the nails.

Here are some worthwhile tips on how to care for your hands using natural remedies which are simple and inexpensive to prepare:

* Clean ingrained dirt and stains or garden-soiled hands by dipping them in warm almond oil, then rubbing them with a mixture of coarse sea salt and equal quantities of dried sage and dried chamomile — enough to form a paste.

* Keep a small bowl of fine bran near the kitchen sink or laundry tub. Dip your hands in the bran and rub thoroughly to cleanse them — instead of over-using soap, which can be drying — then rinse off.

* Soak dried-out hands in warm almond oil, to which has been added 2 drops of carrot oil, for half an hour.

* To strengthen nails, soak them in water to which has been added 1 tablespoon of cider vinegar.

* To clean stained nails, particularly if you smoke, simply paint lemon juice onto them twice a day, using a small paintbrush.

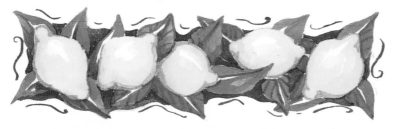

Arms and Elbows

Soaking in the bath presents a great opportunity to take care of arms and elbows. Regular exfoliation of arms with a loofah or loofah mitt will improve the circulation and get rid of dead cells which clog the pores and have a dulling effect on the skin.

Scrub your elbows daily with a soapy pumice stone, or a bath bag filled with oatmeal until all ingrained dirt has disappeared. Next, bleach the reddened skin with lemon juice and finish with a lavish helping of *Massage Moisturising Lotion.*

MASSAGE MOISTURISING LOTION

After exfoliation, massage this lotion into the skin. Use firm strokes, and keep massaging until all traces of the lotion have disappeared.

80 ml (2½ fl oz) almond oil
40 ml (1⅓ fl oz) apricot oil
80 ml (2½ fl oz) glycerine
20 ml (⅔ fl oz) aloe vera juice
5 ml (⅙ fl oz) lemon juice
4 drops pumpkin oil
6 drops chamomile oil

Combine all ingredients in an airtight amber-coloured glass bottle, and shake well until thoroughly blended. Store in a dark, cool place.

Legs

'Thigh flab' and 'cellulite' are both terms used to describe the ugly, rippled bulges which can appear on the inside and back of the thighs. Swimming, dancing, cycling and yoga exercises are all recommended for keeping the leg muscles in trim, which can help control cellulite.

Friction massage with a loofah during a warm bath is also good for accelerating cell metabolism and improving the circulation. Using coarse sea salt on the loofah helps improve skin colour, and is excellent for clearing flaking skin and spots. Always massage in the direction of the heart.

Lower legs can also suffer from flabby muscles, as well as flaky skin and superfluous hair. Dead skin accumulates if your legs are usually clothed in jeans or tight nylon stockings and seldom exposed to the air.

As with the thighs, exfoliating the lower legs with a loofah should be done each time you take a bath. Deal with the more stubborn areas with the addition of coarse sea salt or an oatmeal bath bag; rinse off thoroughly, then massage with the following moisturising cream:

LEG MOISTURISING CREAM
60 g (2 oz) anhydrous lanolin
60 ml (2 fl oz) olive oil
60 ml (2 fl oz) apricot oil

Melt the lanolin and oils together in a double saucepan over low heat. Blend thoroughly, then pour the mixture into a sterilised glass jar with a tight-fitting lid. Let the mixture cool, then seal the jar.

Massage this cream into feet, legs and knees, smoothing it firmly upwards.

Leg Hair

Bathtime can also be used to remove any unwanted leg hair. You can use an electric razor or a hand-held wet razor, both of which leave a bristly stubble after a day or two. If you do use these methods, make sure you moisturise thoroughly with the *Leg Moisturising Cream* after you have finished.

Waxing is a far better method, since hair removed by this process regrows in a weakened state, so that eventually it becomes less necessary to remove it.

HOME-MADE WAX
juice of 2 lemons
500 g (16 oz) white sugar
7 ml (¼ fl oz) glycerine

Melt the sugar in the lemon juice over gentle heat. Cook gently for about 10 minutes until it turns a golden colour. Remove mixture from heat and add glycerine, mixing thoroughly. Use mixture as soon as it has cooled to a comfortable temperature.

Spread the mixture over leg hair, then press a strip of cotton material against it. Draw the cloth towards you, against the direction of the hair growth, so both the wax and hair are removed. When you have finished, rinse legs clean and apply a moisturiser.

Breasts

For women, looking after your breasts is as important as cleansing and moisturising the rest of your body. Too often, they are just soaped and washed — special attention needs to be paid to this delicate area. Gentle massage with an aromatherapy oil blend will aid in toning and firming the breast muscles and smoothing the skin.

Under a hot shower, massage the breasts with strong, firm strokes, pressing upwards from beneath, and continuing over the nipples and up to the chin. After showering, while the skin is still warm and slightly moist, apply a few drops of warm *Breast Massage Oil*. Rotate both palms in small circular movements from the outer sides of each breast in towards the centre, and then upwards from beneath, over the nipples and up to the bottom of the chin.

BREAST MASSAGE OIL
2 drops lavender oil
2 drops rose oil
2 drops geranium oil
20 ml (⅔ fl oz) almond oil

Mix all oils together thoroughly in an egg cup or other small ceramic cup and use as directed.

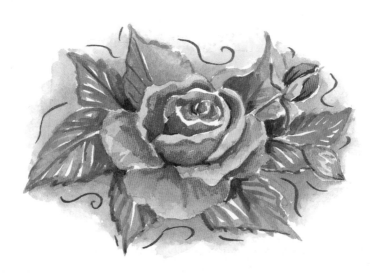

Hot Tubs, Saunas and Steam Rooms

Hot tubs, saunas, steam rooms and whirlpools provide excellent ways to relax and soothe both body and soul after a vigorous workout or a hard day at work. If you have one at home, they also provide an excellent venue for socialising.

Each method has its own advantages: lying back in your own hot tub or jacuzzi, with warm water bubbling over you is much more pleasant than a dip in the chemical-laden stews found in commercial premises. The whirlpool jets of the jacuzzi gently massage your whole body to ease muscle soreness; in addition, essential oils can calm and soothe frazzled nerves, or simply set the mood for more enjoyable activities.

Dry sauna heat lets you sweat off water, while steam heat warms the body quickly, then helps it retain heat to relax tight muscles or soothe sore joints. Saunas are extremely useful for eliminating toxins from the body, but they can leave you feeling a little drained unless you drink water or other fluids. The same applies to steam rooms. The use of essential oils in the sauna will promote the elimination of waste products and debris through the skin. Use them in the water that you throw on the heat source (usually coals).

All these methods have risks, both for healthy people and for those who suffer from heart or blood pressure problems. The greatest problem that confronts ordinarily healthy people who use communal facilities is poor maintenance. This can lead to the spread of skin bacteria and viral or fungal infections. Those with heart problems may be affected by the sudden temperature changes — each time you go from hot to cold, or back again, your heart rate increases by 60% or more, as much as for moderate exercise. As you acclimatise to higher temperatures your blood pressure drops. This could present a risk to people over 50 years of age who are predisposed to arteriosclerosis or have a poorly functioning heart, for such a decline in blood pressure could bring on a mild stroke.

So, before you jump right in and relax in your own private spa, or make use of any of these alternative therapies:

 * *Consider your general state of health and your skin type.*

 * *If you work out vigorously first it may not be wise to risk further water loss.*

 * *When using saunas, novices should limit exposure to 6 minutes or less, and veterans to no more than 15 minutes. Get out immediately if you feel faint.*

* *Drink plenty of water afterwards to replace lost fluids.*

* *Shower and shampoo thoroughly to remove residual salts, acids, metals or chemicals, and moisturise your skin. The* Massage Moisturising Lotion *on page 34 is excellent for this.*

* *People with serious medical problems such as diabetes, vascular problems, hypertension, obesity, kidney dysfunction or metabolic conditions, or who are on daily medication should consult their doctor first.*

* *During pregnancy, it is best to avoid extended periods of heat, especially in the early months.*

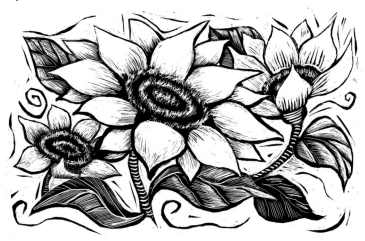

Jacuzzis

Essential oils have been used as aphrodisiacs ever since romance came into being. Why not add them to your jacuzzi and share the scented water with someone special?

The following oils will help enhance a romantic evening. Add them, drop by drop, in the following proportions until the water is sufficiently scented.

3 drops ylang-ylang oil
2 drops rose oil

Or, show your appreciation of your partner by giving him or her a romantic massage. Blend the following essential oils with 30 ml (1 fl oz) of grapeseed oil:

10 drops jasmine oil
10 drops mandarin oil
5 drops black pepper oil
5 drops nutmeg oil

THERAPEUTIC BLENDS

Use whichever combination for *Therapeutic Baths* (see page 24) suits your particular needs. Add the oils a drop at a time, until water is sufficiently scented.

Saunas

Any of the following essential oils can be used singly in the sauna:

EUCALYPTUS • PINE • CYPRESS • ROSEMARY • LEMON • LAVENDER
NIAOULI • LIME • GRAPEFRUIT • BERGAMOT

Add 3 to 6 drops of your selected oil to each cup (250 ml/8 fl oz) of water, and sprinkle this over your heat source.

SINUS BLEND

2 drops basil oil
2 drops lavender oil
2 drops eucalyptus oil
2 drops peppermint oil

Mix the oils together in a cup (250 ml/8 fl oz) of water, and sprinkle this over your heat source.

HEAD COLD

2 drops pine oil
2 drops eucalyptus oil
2 drops cypress oil

Use as for *Sinus Blend.*

STIMULATING AND INVIGORATING

6 drops lavender oil
2 drops rosewood oil
2 drops tangerine oil

Mix the three oils together, then add 4 drops of the mixture to a cup (250ml/8 fl oz) of water and sprinkle this over your heat source.

RELAXING
2 drops geranium oil
3 drops rose oil
5 drops lavender oil

Prepare and use as for *Stimulating and Invigorating Blend.*

DID YOU KNOW . . . ?

That ancient Roman soldiers used the herb rosemary extensively as a bath herb? They would add it to their baths to relieve tired limbs after a long, gruelling march; after a battle, they included bay leaves.

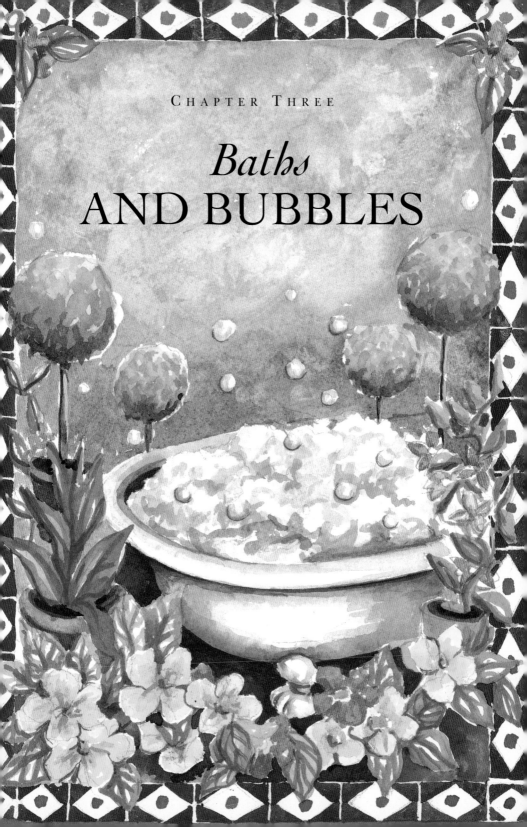

CHAPTER THREE

Baths
AND BUBBLES

Bath Bags

When dried herbs and flowers are held under running water, their beneficial properties and scents are released. Place them in bath bags — see Chapter Two — and hang them from the hot tap, so the water can gush through them while the bath fills. Alternatively, simply drop a bag into the bath and let it bob underneath the jet of water from the tap.

Fill your bath bag with your favourite dried herb or flower, or try the following combinations. Oatmeal has been added to these recipes so that as you use the bag to scrub your body, it will also help soften the skin. Each recipe will provide enough filling for 8 bath bags. Store any leftover mix in an airtight glass jar until required.

ROSEMARY AND MINT MIX
30 g (1 oz) rosemary
15 g (½ oz) peppermint
100 g (3½ oz) coarse oatmeal

SOFT, FRAGRANT MIX
30 g (1 oz) rose petals
30 g (1 oz) lavender buds
15 g (½ oz) thyme
100 g (3½ oz) coarse oatmeal

Washing Bags and Bath Mitts

A washing bag is a herbal bath bag which has been stitched on only two sides, with a drawstring on the top. The addition of dried soapwort to the herb mix will give a gentle cleansing effect. Oatmeal may also be included to remove any dead skin cells, and so can lovage, which is mildly antiseptic and excellent for cleansing spotty skin, as well as acting as a mild deodorant.

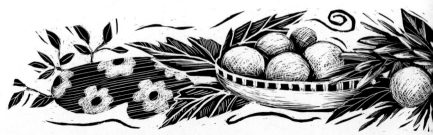

Bath mitts add a touch of luxury to your bath, and also make attractive and unusual gifts. They are simple to make, too. To make your mitt you will need:

a piece of towelling 25 x 45 cm (10 x 18 in)
brown paper for pattern
sewing thread
15 cm (6 in) of velcro, cut into two 7.5cm (3 in) pieces

Cut the towelling into three 25 x 15 cm (10 x 6 in) pieces. Stack the pieces on top of one another.

Place your hand on the brown paper and draw around it. Cut out the shape, leaving a straight edge at the wrist — this is the pattern for your mitt.

Cut a mitt shape from each towelling piece. Fold a 1 cm (½ in) hem in on the wrong side of the straight edge of each mitt piece. Stitch the hem down on one piece. Stitch velcro across the remaining folded raw hems on the wrong side. Press the velcro strips together. Place mitt with hemmed edge over the velcro-trimmed pieces with right sides facing. Stitch around the sides and top. Turn to right side.

Fillings

Use only dried herbs and flowers and mix all ingredients together thoroughly. Each recipe will make enough filling for 3 mitts or 4 bags. Store any leftover mixture in an airtight glass jar for future use.

CHAMOMILE AND LAVENDER
30 g (1 oz) chamomile
30 g (1 oz) lavender
15 g (½ oz) soapwort
100 g (3½ oz) almond meal

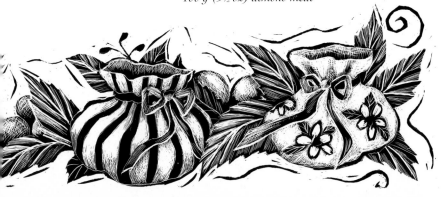

PEPPERMINT AND ELDER FLOWER

30 g (1 oz) peppermint
30 g (1 oz) elder flowers
10 g (⅓ oz) soapwort
100 g (3½ oz) almond meal

SWEET AMBROSIA

40 g (1½ oz) rose petals
30 g (1 oz) lavender
15 g (½ oz) lovage root
100 g (3½ oz) almond meal

Soapy Bags

Make your soapy bag slightly larger than a washing bag or bath bag.

Take a 25 cm (10 in) square of muslin. Mix together 2 tablespoons of dried herbs of your choice, 2 tablespoons of medium oatmeal, and 1 tablespoon of grated, unscented, pure soap. Place the oatmeal and soap in the middle of the muslin, draw up the sides and tie with ribbon. Use the bag to gently wash and massage your body.

CORNMEAL WASHING BAG

Make this bag thin and flat so that it can be used as a washing mitt. Fill with a mixture of equal parts cornmeal and dried herbs of your choice.

Place the bag over your hand and gently scrub your body, paying particular attention to heels, knees and elbows. The cornmeal will help cleanse the skin and remove any dead cells.

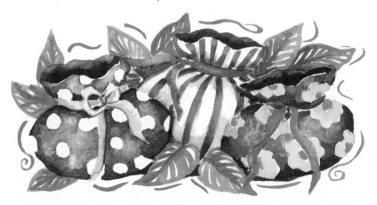

Wash Balls

POTPOURRI WASH BALLS

These delightfully fragrant soap balls are attractive in any bathroom and are suitable for all skin types. Tie them up in muslin bags for use as a type of soapy sponge.

5 cups dried scented geranium leaves
3 cups dried lavender buds
3 cups dried rose petals
2 cups (310 g/ 10 oz) pure soap, coarsely grated
2 cups (310 g/ 10 oz) large oat flakes (not instant)
geranium oil

Combine dried herbs with the soap and oats. Add a few drops of geranium oil, 1 drop at a time, until the mixture is sufficiently scented. Seal in an airtight glass jar and allow to mature for 1 week. Mix again, form into balls and put into the muslin bags. This mixture will make approximately 12 wash balls.

To make your bags, cut 10 cm (4 in) squares of muslin, place a ball in each one, draw up the sides and tie with a piece of ribbon. These make an unusual and attractive gift for Christmas or other special occasions.

Herbal Wash Balls

A jar of aromatic soap washballs makes a lovely gift. Or keep them for when you feel like spoiling yourself with a fragrant treat.

FLORAL WASH BALLS

310 g (10 oz) pure white soap, grated
310 ml (10 fl oz) rose-water
10 drops oil of cloves
3 tablespoons dried lavender
3 tablespoons dried rose petals
2 tablespoons dried marjoram

Put the grated soap in a large ceramic mixing bowl. Heat 250 ml (8 fl oz) of rose-water to just below boiling point and pour it over the soap. Blend the mixture thoroughly with a wooden spoon, then let it stand for

10 minutes. Knead it with your hands to make a smooth paste, then mix in the oil of cloves and the dried herbs. Leave in a warm spot for 10 minutes or until the soap begins to dry and becomes pliable. Form the soap into small balls about the size of a golf ball, and leave them in the sun (on a sheet of plastic wrap) for about 2 hours to firm up.

Moisten your hands with the remaining rose-water and rub the balls to make them smooth and shiny, then put them back on the plastic wrap and leave them in a warm spot for 24 hours to firm completely.

For gift giving, package the wash balls in a pretty net or organza bag, or a glass jar decorated with coloured ribbon and lace.

Other Fragrances

You can mix and blend dried herbs and essential oils to make a delightful range of aromatic soap wash balls. Try the following oil and herb blends, preparing them with the same quantities of grated soap and floral water as in the recipe above.

LEMON DELIGHT

2 ml (⅟₁₂ fl oz) lemon oil
3 drops bergamot oil
orange flower water
3 tablespoons dried lemon verbena
3 tablespoons dried marjoram

CITRUS MINT

2 ml (⅟₁₂ fl oz) lemon oil
4 drops peppermint oil
orange flower water
3 tablespoons dried peppermint
3 tablespoons dried geranium (preferably
the spicy variety — P. denticulatum)

MYSTIC AMBROSIA

10 drops rose oil
4 drops clove oil
4 drops cinnamon oil
3 tablespoons dried rose petals
2 tablespoons dried lavender

EXOTIC NIGHTS

20 drops lavender oil
6 drops sandalwood oil
rose-water
3 tablespoons dried lavender
3 tablespoons dried rose petals
2 tablespoons dried marjoram

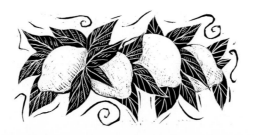

Soap for all Occasions

Making soap from scratch is a time-consuming and complicated business and with most people today having very busy lives, it is far from practical. However, 'personalised' herbal soaps made from a base of pure, unperfumed soap are easy and fun to make. You can also add honey or oatmeal and therapeutic and fragrant herbs. These soaps will cleanse and rinse away dirt just as effectively as commercially available ones, and will also exert their beneficial effects on the outer layer of the skin — the so-called 'horny' or epithelial layer — making it smooth and soft.

ROSE PETAL SOAP

This pure, mild, and fragrant blend is particularly suitable for babies.

Put 10 tablespoons of finely grated Castille soap (from the chemist) in a saucepan, cover with water and soak for 24 hours, giving an occasional stir.

Crush 2 tablespoons of dried rose petals and reduce them to a powder by rubbing through a fine wire sieve; set aside.

Bring the soap mixture to the boil, stirring until it is dissolved. Remove from the heat, add 1 tablespoon of almond oil for each cupful, plus the powdered rose petals, and stir thoroughly to blend. Add essential oil of rose, drop by drop, until sufficiently scented. Pour mixture into moulds and allow to harden for 2 weeks before using.

Moulds can be small, shallow cardboard containers, patty pans, chocolate moulds, circles, triangles — anything you can think of. Interesting shapes will make bath time fun for the kids. You can also display the soap in a glass jar or on an attractive ceramic dish, as a bathroom feature.

CHAMOMILE SOAP

A gentle emollient soap that is suitable for all skin types; this blend is also healing and soothing for disturbed skin.

5 tablespoons dried chamomile
310 ml (10 fl oz) boiling water
350 g (11½ oz) pure, unscented grated soap

Put the chamomile in a ceramic bowl and add the boiling water. Cover and infuse for 12 hours then strain through muslin cloth, squeezing out all the liquid.

Prepare soap base as for *Rose Petal Soap*, add chamomile infusion, and stir thoroughly to blend.

YARROW SOAP

This is an excellent soap for oily skins, as it helps regulate over-active sebaceous glands.

3 tablespoons dried yarrow
310 ml (10 fl oz) boiling water
350 g (11½ oz) pure, unscented grated soap

Infuse herbs as for *Chamomile Soap*, then continue as for *Rose Petal Soap*.

CALENDULA SOAP

Use this whenever you need a medicated soap. It is especially suitable for inflamed skin.

25 g (1 oz) marshmallow root
25 g (1 oz) malva leaf
1 litre (32 fl oz) distilled water
350 g (11½ oz) pure, unscented grated soap
5 tablespoons dried calendula petals

Chop up the marshmallow root and put it in an enamel or stainless steel pan with the malva leaf and the distilled water. Bring to the boil and then simmer for 15 minutes. Remove from heat, add the calendula petals, cover and steep for 8 hours. Strain through muslin and add to *Rose Petal Soap* recipe. Continue as for *Rose Petal Soap*.

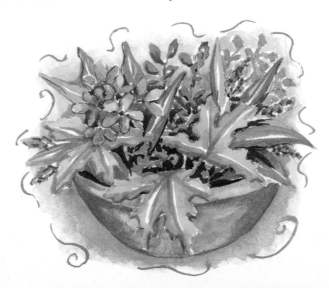

OATMEAL SOAP

Oatmeal has a soothing and smoothing effect on the skin.

450 g (14 oz) pure, unscented grated soap
250 ml (8 oz) chamomile infusion
225 g (7 oz) oatmeal

Prepare the soap as for *Rose Petal Soap*, stirring in the oatmeal just before pouring the soap into moulds.

ALMOND SOAP

This is a soothing soap substitute that is particularly good for gently cleansing sunburnt skin. Use a tablespoonful at a time, smoothing it on as you would a face pack. Leave for a few minutes before washing off.

2 tablespoons finely-ground almonds
2 tablespoons kaolin or china clay (available from the chemist)
almond oil, sufficient
rose-water, sufficient

Mix all the ingredients together, adding sufficient and equal quantities of almond oil and rose-water to form a stiff paste. Store in a jar with a tight-fitting lid.

ROSE MOISTURISING SOAP

This is an excellent emollient soap which will leave your skin feeling smooth and soft, and moisturise it at the same time.

2 cups (310 g/10 oz) grated soap
2 tablespoons honey
2 tablespoons anhydrous lanolin
20 ml (⅔ fl oz) almond oil
15 ml (½ fl oz) rose-water
5 ml (⅙ fl oz) essential oil of rose
water, sufficient

Put the grated soap in a saucepan, cover with water and leave to soak for 24 hours, giving an occasional stir.

Bring the soap mixture to the boil in a double saucepan, then reduce to a gentle simmer, stirring continuously while it dissolves. When mixture is almost completely melted, add the honey and anhydrous lanolin, continuing to stir until well blended. Remove from heat and stir in the almond oil, rose-water and rose oil.

Pour mixture into moulds and allow to harden for 2 weeks before using.

HERBAL SOAP GEL

An ideal soap that will make bath time fun for the kids. Keep this jelly-like soap in a large container by the bath; it's ideal for washing hands, too.

2 teaspoons dried lemon verbena
2 teaspoons dried rosemary
2 teaspoons dried sage
2 teaspoons dried thyme
15 g (½ oz) grated soap
2¼ litres (72 fl oz) water

Put the herbs in a large ceramic bowl and add 1 litre (32 fl oz) of the boiling water. Cover and allow to steep overnight. Then strain through muslin, squeezing all liquid from the herbs.

Add the grated soap and a little of the reserved water to a saucepan. Bring mixture to the boil, stirring constantly until the soap has dissolved (use a potato masher, if necessary). Boil the remainder of the water and combine it with the soap solution and herbal infusion in a large bowl, stirring until well blended. Leave until it sets into a soft gel and then store in an airtight container.

SOAPWORT AND LIME FLOWER WASHING LATHER

Half a cup of this fragrant liquid added to bath water will have a gentle, cleansing effect and leave the skin feeling smooth and soft rather than 'dried out', as so often happens with commercial soaps.

40 g (1½ oz) dried soapwort
1 litre (32 fl oz) distilled water
20 g (⅔ oz) dried lime flowers

Put the soapwort and distilled water in an enamel or stainless steel saucepan, bring to the boil and gently simmer for 15 minutes. Remove mixture from heat, add lime flowers, cover and steep overnight. Strain through muslin, squeezing all liquid from the herbs. Store in an airtight bottle in a cool spot.

FRAGRANT SHOWER GEL

Rub this gel over your body, while showering, for a gentle cleansing effect that leaves the skin feeling soft and smooth.

40 g (1½ oz) dried soapwort
625 ml (20 fl oz) distilled water
3 teaspoons dried fragrant herb of choice
15 ml (½ fl oz) vodka
arrowroot

Put the soapwort and distilled water in an enamel or stainless steel pan, bring to the boil and gently boil for 15 minutes. Remove from heat, add the herbs, cover, steep for 8 hours and strain through muslin.

After straining, measure the liquid, return to the saucepan, add the vodka and 2 teaspoons of powdered arrowroot to every 80 ml (2½ fl oz) of liquid. Heat gently, and stir continuously, until the mixture thickens and clears. Remove from heat and store in a wide-mouthed, airtight container.

Bubble Baths

NOURISHING BUBBLE BATH OIL

This is a nourishing and softening bath oil for all the family. It is ideal for those times when you just feel like relaxing and luxuriating in a warm bubble bath.

2 teaspoons each of dried chamomile, dried rosemary and dried lime flowers
1 litre (35 fl oz) boiling water
1 cup (155 g/5 oz) pure white soap, grated
15 ml (½ fl oz) wheatgerm oil
50 ml (2 fl oz) glycerine
few drops of lime oil
25 ml (1 fl oz) witch-hazel

Put the dried herbs in a ceramic bowl and add the boiling water. Cover, steep for 12 hours and strain through muslin.

Dissolve the soap in the herbal infusion in an enamel or stainless steel saucepan over a medium heat, stirring continuously. Put the wheatgerm oil, glycerine, essential oil and witch-hazel in a bowl and whisk until well blended. Add the dissolved soap mixture and beat with an electric mixer until the mixture is thoroughly emulsified. Store in a bottle with a tight-fitting lid.

Add a teaspoonful to the bath water while the taps are running.

BUBBLE BATH LIQUID FOR KIDS

This is a great way for kids to enjoy their bath, while they wash away dirt and grime.

fragrant, dried herb of choice
310 ml (10 fl oz) soft water, boiling
10 g (⅓ oz) pure white soap, grated
50 ml (2 fl oz) glycerine

Put 2 teaspoons of fragrant herb in a ceramic bowl with the boiling water. Cover, steep for 3 hours, strain through muslin, squeezing all liquid from the herbs, and add required amount to recipe.

Add the grated soap and herb water to an enamel pan and stir continually over a medium heat until the soap has completely dissolved. Stir in the glycerine until well blended, remove from heat, cool, and store in a tightly capped bottle.

Pour a small amount into the bath while the taps are running, swishing around to create the bubbles.

FRAGRANT BATH SALTS

These can be expensive to buy, yet are easily made at home. When you feel like pampering yourself, just add a couple of handfuls of these bath salts to your bath — and then luxuriate!

560 g (18 oz) bicarbonate of soda
15 g (½ oz) dried lavender
7 ml (¼ fl oz) rosemary oil
7 ml (¼ fl oz) eucalyptus oil

Thoroughly mix all ingredients together and store in an airtight jar.

To use, place 2 handfuls of the mixture in the centre of a muslin square, draw up the sides and tie with a piece of ribbon. Swirl the bag around in the bath water until contents are completely dissolved. When you have finished soaking, rub the muslin bag gently over your body until the scent of the lavender is exhausted.

DID YOU KNOW . . . ?

That natural herb soaps exert their effect on the outer layer of the skin
— the so-called 'horny' or epithelial layer — making it smooth and soft.

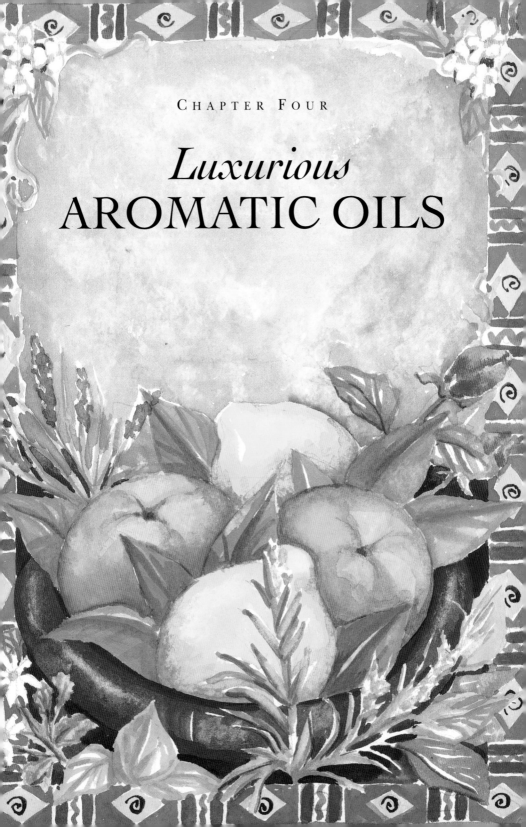

CHAPTER FOUR

Luxurious
AROMATIC OILS

Nourishing Bath Oils

Adding aromatic oils to your bath water will fill the bathroom with a wonderful fragrance, as well as leaving your skin silky-textured.

Although there is a huge variety of commercial bath oils available, it is far more rewarding and satisfying to make your own special blends. You can either simply combine a few drops of pure essential oils each time you take a bath, or blend them with a base oil such as almond, avocado or sunflower oil. You can also use treated castor oil, sometimes referred to as turkey red oil, which is a pure, odourless oil that will disperse easily in water.

To make a bath oil, dilute 50 drops of your chosen essential oil or mixed blend in 50 ml (2 fl oz) of base oil. Shake well, and add about 10 drops of oil to the bath water while the taps are running.

Bath Oils to Try

The following essential oils will provide you with an excellent 'wardrobe' of bath scents for most situations. Start with a few oils, depending on your immediate needs or circumstances, then add more as you become familiar with the various herbs and their beneficial properties.

ESSENTIAL OIL	BENEFICIAL EFFECT
BASIL	*Refreshing, uplifting, stimulating, invigorating, energising and anti-depressant; do not use more than 3 drops of neat oil in the bath — it may irritate some skin types.*
BAY LEAF	*Very aromatic; soothing to the senses and comforting to tired and aching limbs.*
BERGAMOT	*Fresh, aromatic, uplifting, antiseptic, relaxing and an inducement to restful sleep; do not use neat; use no more than 0.5 to 1% concentration in the base oil.*
CHAMOMILE	*Very soothing, relaxing, calming and comforting to the nerves; an inducement to sound natural sleep.*
CYPRESS	*Refreshing, stimulating and invigorating.*
EUCALYPTUS	*Highly aromatic; refreshing, head-clearing (clears a stuffy nose so you can breathe more easily); anti-viral; relieves muscular pain.*
FRANKINCENSE	*Warming and relaxing; considered rejuvenating.*
GERANIUM (ALL TYPES)	*Very aromatic, refreshing and relaxing.*
GINGER	*Stimulating tonic; valuable bath oil to ward off colds.*

HYSSOP	*Relieves stiffness from overwork or sport; use only in moderation as it can be toxic. Do not use if you are an epileptic.*
JASMINE	*Soothing and relaxing, sedative; has a powerful fragrance.*
LAVENDER	*Refreshing aromatic scent; relaxing, soothing, calming and a natural disinfectant; low toxicity makes it good for children.*
LEMONGRASS	*Refreshing, reviving, revitalising, uplifting, toning and antiseptic; helps heal skin complaints.*
LIME FLOWER	*Very calming.*
LOVAGE	*Relaxing and rejuvenating, with natural deodorant properties.*
MARJORAM	*Aromatic; calming, warming and fortifying.*
NEROLI	*Ambrosial and heady scent; very calming; antiseptic; excellent for skin.*
ORANGE	*Refreshing, reviving and restoring.*
PATCHOULI	*Exotic perfume; very relaxing and comforting; antiseptic and antidepressant. Small quantities are uplifting; large doses are sedative.*
PEPPERMINT	*Extra invigorating and antiseptic; a comforting, satisfying and refreshing scent that clears the head and improves breathing. Use at a low concentration (1%) on inflamed or sensitive skin.*
PINE	*Extra invigorating, with a clean, refreshing scent; reviving, stimulating, antiseptic and disinfectant.*
ROSE	*Relaxing, calming, antidepressant and antiseptic; softens the skin, one of the least toxic oils — good for children.*
ROSEMARY	*Refreshing aromatic scent; toning, stimulating and invigorating; relieves stiff joints and relaxes aching muscles.*
ROSEWOOD	*Uplifting, stimulating and invigorating.*
SAGE	*Aromatic; soothing, refreshing, relaxing and enlivening. Use in moderation as it can be toxic. Do not use if breastfeeding. Clary sage is also comforting and satisfying and reputed to be an aphrodisiac. Use sparingly — even small percentages may induce intoxication and large percentages may induce headaches.*
SANDALWOOD	*Calming, relaxing and uplifting; antiseptic.*
TANGERINE	*Stimulating and invigorating; helps improve energy levels.*
TEA TREE	*Powerful antiseptic and fungicide — highly disinfectant without being toxic; toning and head-clearing.*
THYME	*Delightful aromatic scent; natural antiseptic and deodorant; stimulating.*
YLANG-YLANG	*Calming, comforting and satisfying; sedative, antiseptic and antidepressant. Use sparingly — too much may cause headaches.*

Fragrant Bath Blends

Plain old tap-water can sometimes have a very drying effect on the skin. The addition of a bath oil will help counteract this. Mix your own special blends or choose from any of the following recipes:

ROSE NOURISHING BATH OIL

This bath blend will nourish and soften the skin, while helping soothe, calm and relax the body and mind at the same time.

15 ml (½ fl oz) avocado oil
10 ml (⅓ fl oz) apricot kernel oil
25 ml (1 fl oz) almond oil
35 drops rose oil
10 drops lavender oil
5 drops chamomile oil

Blend the base oils thoroughly, then add the essential oils, blending well. Store in an airtight, amber-coloured glass bottle away from sunlight and direct heat.

CITRUS BATH OIL

Use this oil for a refreshing and invigorating bath. It is a great pick-me-up first thing in the morning.

50 ml (2 fl oz) base oil
35 drops lemon oil
15 drops orange oil
5 drops lime oil

SPICY BATH OIL

An exotic, aromatic blend that will transport your mind and soul to the ancient land of *The Arabian Nights*. Ideal when romance is on your mind and you're in the mood to share your bath with that special someone!

50 ml (2 fl oz) base oil
8 drops cypress oil
8 drops sandalwood oil
34 drops clove oil

Therapeutic Bath Blends

DRY SKIN

A nourishing oil blend, very useful for those who suffer from dry and flaky skin.

50 ml (2 fl oz) almond oil
6 drops palma rosa oil
16 drops rose oil
10 drops carrot oil
8 drops German chamomile oil

OILY SKIN

50 ml (2 fl oz) base oil
20 drops lemon oil
15 drops sandalwood oil
10 drops cypress oil
5 drops ylang-ylang oil

SENSITIVE SKIN

45 ml (1½ fl oz) almond oil
5 ml (⅙ fl oz) avocado oil
30 drops rose oil
10 drops sandalwood oil
5 drops neroli oil
5 drops chamomile oil

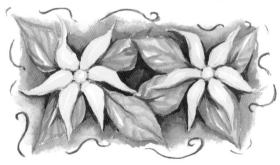

STRESS

This aromatic blend will help you relax and unwind at the end of a busy day. Use it whenever you feel the need to bring body and soul back into perfect harmony.

45 ml (1½ fl oz) almond oil
5 ml (⅙ fl oz) wheatgerm oil
25 drops rose oil
10 drops lavender oil
10 drops sandalwood oil
5 drops ylang-ylang oil

MENTAL FATIGUE

50 ml (2 fl oz) base oil
40 drops rosemary oil
7 drops peppermint oil
3 drops basil oil

IRRITABILITY

50 ml (2 fl oz) base oil
30 drops lavender oil
15 drops neroli oil
5 drops chamomile oil

APHRODISIAC BATH OIL

When sharing a bath — and then bed — is all that is on your mind, this aphrodisiac oil blend will set the mood for passion and enjoyment.

50 ml (2 fl oz) base oil
25 drops rose oil
15 drops sandalwood oil
4 drops ylang-ylang oil
3 drops clary sage oil

After the bath, give each other a romantic and relaxing massage with the following oil blend:

30 ml (1 fl oz) grapeseed oil
10 drops rose oil
10 drops palma rosa oil
2 drops ylang-ylang oil
8 drops lemon oil

Dilute the essential oils in the carrier oil in a ceramic egg cup, or other suitable vessel.

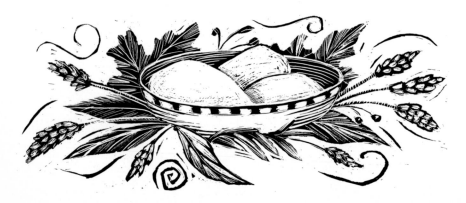

DEPRESSING MOODS

Add 50 drops of any of the following essential oils (either just one or a mixture), to 50 ml (2 fl oz) of base oil to ease these moods:

MELANCHOLY   *rose, neroli or chamomile*
ANXIETY   *chamomile, neroli or lavender*
ANGER   *rose or chamomile*

Herbal Bath Oils

Herbal bath oils are made by steeping fresh herbs in a base oil such as those used for the essential oil blends.

Choose three or four good handfuls of a favourite herb or herbs, or any of those listed in Chapter One. Spread them out on a shallow, flat tray and sprinkle a quantity of non-iodised salt over, enough to cover them. Place a layer of the salted herbs in a wide-mouthed glass jar and then a layer of cottonwool, combed out thinly and soaked in a suitable base oil. For moisturising oils, choose almond oil as the carrier. Repeat this procedure, alternating layers of herbs and oiled cottonwool until the jar is full. Seal with a piece of plastic wrap and leave in a sunny spot for at least 15 days, then squeeze the fragrant oil from the whole mass. Strain oil and store it in an airtight, amber-coloured glass bottle. A tablespoon of wheatgerm oil added to the jar before you seal it will act as a natural preservative.

Use sparingly — 1 to 2 tablespoonfuls — in the bath.

SOOTHING BATH OIL

This herbal bath oil will soothe, smooth and nourish the skin. It is easily made by steeping fragrant rose petals in oil. Choose a 1¼ litre (2 pint) glass jar and fill with as many petals as possible. Combine the following oils as the carrier:

500 ml (16 fl oz) almond oil
250 ml (8 fl oz) sunflower oil
125 ml (4 fl oz) wheatgerm oil

Steep petals until oil is sufficiently fragrant. When you strain the fragrant oil, add a few drops of essential oil of rose, a drop at a time, to adjust the scent to your liking.

CALENDULA SKIN SOFTENER

Use this herbal bath oil to soften the skin and help heal cracking and chapping.

calendula petals, sufficient
500 ml (16 fl oz) almond oil
50 ml (2 fl oz) wheatgerm oil
50 ml (2 fl oz) avocado oil
few drops of favourite essential oil

Prepare as for *Soothing Bath Oil.*

Pre-bath Body Oils

Although the usual practice is to apply body oils after a bath or shower, it is also tremendously satisfying to apply them beforehand. As the oil comes into contact with the water, you will feel as though you are completely enveloped in scent. As a bonus the oil is more readily absorbed into the skin by osmosis. Choose from any of the essential oils listed previously, and use them, singly or in combination, to suit your particular mood.

As with the bath oils, the essential oils should first be diluted in a suitable base, such as almond oil. Add 1 drop of essential oil to every millilitre of base oil, then dilute the mixture 50:50 with water and rub over your entire body. To make the base oil extra nourishing and penetrating, prepare the recipe that follows before adding the essential oils:

25 ml (1 fl oz) almond oil
5 ml (⅙ fl oz) avocado oil
20 drops jojoba oil
5 drops carrot oil

This base is nourishing and is an excellent emollient, being rich in protein and vitamins. It will leave your skin with a satiny smooth feeling.

Suggested Blends

SOFTENING
20 drops rose oil
5 drops frankincense oil
5 drops lavender oil

RELAXING
20 drops rose oil
5 drops neroli oil
5 drops chamomile oil

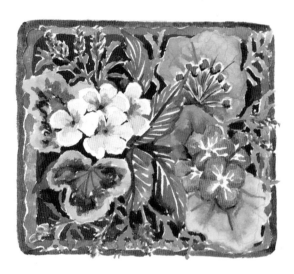

REFINING
15 drops lemongrass oil
10 drops geranium oil
5 drops lavender oil

UPLIFTING
15 drops lemon oil
10 drops lavender oil
5 drops bergamot oil

TONING
10 drops frankincense oil
6 drops rosemary oil
4 drops chamomile oil
6 drops geranium oil
4 drops neroli oil

FATIGUE
10 drops rosemary oil
15 drops geranium oil
3 drops peppermint oil
2 drops basil oil

Body Lotions

Keep your skin looking healthy and supple by pampering it with an after-bath body lotion. Remember, though, herbal skin care preparations alone won't give your body that healthy glow. A holistic approach to your health, which includes regular exercise and a good diet, is essential.

Daily use of a moisturising lotion or cream will help protect your skin by replacing natural oils which are lost through bathing and exposure to the sun.

ROSE AND HONEY BODY LOTION

20 ml (⅔ fl oz) chamomile infusion
80 ml (2½ fl oz) quince gel
125 ml (4 fl oz) almond oil
5 ml (⅙ fl oz) clear honey
4 drops essential oil of rose

To make the chamomile infusion:

Put a level teaspoon of dried chamomile in a ceramic bowl and add 310 ml (10 fl oz) of boiling water. Cover and infuse until cool. Strain through muslin and add required amount to the recipe.

To make the quince gel:

Add 1 teaspoon of seeds from a ripened quince to a saucepan containing 250 ml (8 fl oz) of distilled water. Bring slowly to the boil and simmer gently for about 15 minutes, stirring to prevent sticking. The mixture will thicken into a gel. Strain off the seeds and save in the refrigerator — they can be used several times.

Warm the almond oil and the chamomile infusion in a saucepan over low heat, then stir in honey, until well blended. Remove from heat, allow to cool, then combine with the rest of the ingredients and store in an airtight jar. Shake well to ensure that all ingredients are well mixed.

ROSE-WATER LOTION

55 g (2 oz) anhydrous lanolin
30 ml (1 fl oz) soya oil
25 ml (1 fl oz) almond oil
¼ teaspoon tincture of benzoin
125 ml (4 fl oz) rose-water

Melt the lanolin and oils together in a double saucepan over a medium heat. When completely liquefied and blended, remove from heat and pour into a ceramic bowl. Add tincture of benzoin, then beat at high speed while you add the rose-water in a thin stream. Beat until mixture thickens and becomes creamy. Store in an airtight jar.

INTENSIVE CARE BODY LOTION

This lotion may be used to soothe and repair skin that has become dry and scaly. It will help heal even very damaged skin, keeping it smooth and supple.

100 g (3½ oz) glycerine
5 ml (⅙ fl oz) wheatgerm oil
20 ml (⅔ fl oz) almond oil
10 ml (⅓ fl oz) avocado oil
10 ml (⅓ fl oz) sunflower oil
10 ml (⅓ fl oz) jojoba oil
30 ml (1 fl oz) aloe vera juice
45 ml (1½ fl oz) distilled water
6 drops rose oil
4 drops neroli oil
4 drops chamomile oil
8 drops lemon juice

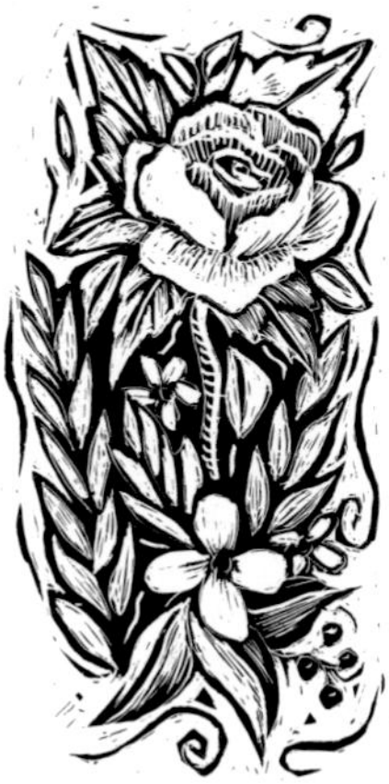

Place all the ingredients in a ceramic bowl and beat vigorously until thoroughly emulsified. Store in an airtight glass bottle in a cool, dark place until needed. Shake well before use.

To apply, massage well into affected areas of skin.

EVERY DAY ROSE BODY MOISTURISER

Use this lotion every day to soothe your skin and keep it feeling smooth and supple.

100 g (3½ oz) glycerine
75 ml (2½ fl oz) rose-water
45 ml (1½ fl oz) almond oil
20 ml (⅔ fl oz) wheatgerm oil
12 drops rose oil
5 ml (⅙ fl oz) jojoba oil
8 drops lemon juice

Prepare as for *Intensive Care Body Lotion.* To apply, massage well into skin.

RICH BODY LOTION

60 ml (2 fl oz) almond oil
20 ml (⅔ fl oz) apricot kernel oil
10 ml (⅓ fl oz) avocado oil
5 ml (⅙ fl oz) jojoba oil
5 ml (⅙ fl oz) wheatgerm oil
35 drops palma rosa oil
40 drops lavender oil
15 drops neroli oil
10 drops frankincense oil

Place all the oils in an amber-coloured glass bottle, seal and shake well to mix. Store away from direct heat and sunlight.

To use, rub generously into skin after bath or shower.

AFTER-BATH DEODORISING OIL

Those who are prone to profuse and unpleasant-smelling perspiration should use this after-bath body oil. Apply the oil generously, rubbing well into the skin.

20 ml (⅔ fl oz) almond oil
5 ml (⅙ fl oz) jojoba oil
5 ml (⅙ fl oz) wheatgerm oil
15 drops lavender oil
10 drops lemongrass oil
5 drops eucalyptus oil

Blend all oils together thoroughly in an airtight, amber-coloured glass bottle. Keep away from direct sunlight and heat.

After-bath Massage

After-bath 'aroma massage' oils are an ideal way to use essential oils to help heal tired, sore and aching muscles, relieve tension and stress, and promote relaxation. You can easily apply them yourself: it is neither difficult nor complicated.

Massage is an effective drugless therapy that enhances circulation and improves skin and muscle tone. Fatigue-producing chemicals are cleared away and the nerve endings of the skin are soothed and relaxed.

The Body

* Pour a teaspoon of oil into your palm, rub your hands together, then apply oil to the breasts and buttocks with a circular motion.

* Using a small amount of additional oil, rub your solar plexus six times in an anti-clockwise direction. Then stroke the residual oil upwards over your stomach, using both hands.

* Put another teaspoon of oil in your palm, rub your hands together, and massage each arm with firm strokes from the hand to the shoulder. Finish off by deeply, yet gently, kneading up the arm with your fingers.

* Using one more teaspoon of oil, work upwards over your legs with deep, firm strokes. Move from the ankle to the top of your thighs, working with both hands.

The Feet

* Place your hand so that your thumb is on the top of your foot and your fingers on the sole. Stroke your thumb down from the ankle to the toes repeatedly, applying firm pressure. Commence circular kneading movements all around the ankle and foot then knead up and down the top part of the foot with your thumbs, pressing the sole from beneath with your fingers.

* Move to the toes and knead each one up and down between your thumb and forefinger. Then place your foot across your knee, and knead your entire sole with your fingers. You will need to use good firm pressure, as the sole is a heavily-padded spot.

* Repeat procedure with other foot.

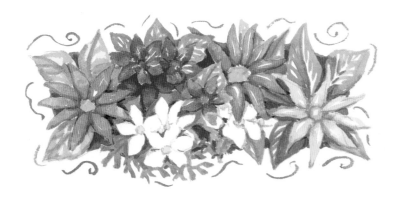

The Face

* Start by placing one hand flat across your forehead, fingers facing to the side. Stroke straight down to the bridge of your nose, immediately replacing the first hand with your other hand, using a smooth, hand-over-hand action.

* Next, place fingers of both hands on forehead so that they meet in the centre. Commence slow, circular, gentle kneading from middle of forehead to temples and sides of head.

* Place one hand on each cheek, and gently massage with a rhythmic, to-and-fro movement, continuing down to the jaw and chin area. Change to a gentle, yet firm, hand-over-hand movement from the base of the neck up to the tip of the chin.

* Move to the mouth and massage muscles firmly, yet gently, by circling lips with your index fingertips. Still using your fingertips, massage areas of the face you haven't yet reached.

Head, Neck and Shoulders

To massage these areas you will need some help from your partner — and what a delightful experience this will be, after you both emerge from a relaxing, aromatic bath!

To fully enjoy the experience, your partner should follow these tips:

* Maintain a constant, even rhythm in your movements.

* Always balance the movements.

* Be aware of any particular tension spots that need special attention.

* Make sure that your partner is kept warm. Cover any area that is not being massaged with a warm towel.

* Focus fully on the massage and on the person being massaged.

* Keep all distractions and interruptions to an absolute minimum.

* Silence is the golden rule — discussion about what is being done will only interfere with full sensual appreciation.

* If receiving the massage, empty your mind of all thoughts. Allow your body to hang loose, limp and relaxed.

TECHNIQUE

* *First, focus on the neck. Place your hands on one side of your partner's neck and make small circular movements with your fingers. Massage along sides and back of neck, from base of skull to shoulders. Repeat movements on other side of neck.*

* *Cradle the base of your partner's skull in both your hands, letting your thumbs hang free. Stroke back and forth on the neck, pressing up against the muscles. Without changing this position, begin to massage the base of their skull with your finger, using a vibrating motion.*

* *Next, place one hand over the top of your partner's head and the other at the base of the skull to support it. Press down with your top hand, moving it back and forth in small circles. Go from the hairline to the back of the head, then gently push the head forward and continue down the back of the neck. Finish massaging the head by kneading the scalp in small circular movements with your fingers. (Do not use oil on the scalp — it is self-lubricating.)*

* *Place your fingertips over the top of your partner's shoulders, with your thumbs sitting on the base of their neck. Begin working your fingertips and thumbs firmly into the muscles, then move over the neck with your thumbs, using a rhythmic, circular, kneading movement. Work well into all tense areas on the sides of the neck.*

Massage Oil Blends

BODY MASSAGE OIL

Towel dry your body immediately after your bath or shower, and apply this smoothing body oil. It is warming, relaxing, nourishing and rejuvenating to the skin.

85 ml (3 fl oz) almond oil
40 ml (1½ fl oz) apricot kernel oil
25 ml (1 fl oz) jojoba oil
60 drops frankincense oil
30 drops neroli oil

Combine all ingredients in an airtight amber-coloured glass bottle. Shake vigorously until all the oils have completely emulsified.

All the massage oil recipes given here are blended in this way.

MUSCULAR ACHES

Use this after-bath body massage oil for tired, sore and aching muscles.

40 ml (1½ fl oz) hazelnut oil
5 ml (⅙ fl oz) avocado oil
5 ml (⅙ fl oz) jojoba oil
8 drops rosemary oil
8 drops bergamot oil
8 drops coriander oil
6 drops eucalyptus oil

STRETCH MARKS

Apply generously, massaging well into problem areas.

40 ml (1½ fl oz) almond oil
5 ml (⅙ fl oz) avocado oil
5 ml (⅙ fl oz) jojoba oil
10 drops frankincense
15 drops lavender oil
5 drops neroli oil

ANTI-CELLULITE

40 ml (1½ fl oz) hazelnut oil
5 ml (⅙ fl oz) avocado oil
5 ml (⅙ fl oz) jojoba oil
8 drops rosemary oil
8 drops fennel oil
8 drops oregano oil

POOR CIRCULATION

40 ml (1½ fl oz) almond oil
5 ml (⅙ fl oz) avocado oil
5 ml (⅙ fl oz) wheatgerm oil
12 drops black pepper oil
12 drops juniper oil
8 drops cypress oil

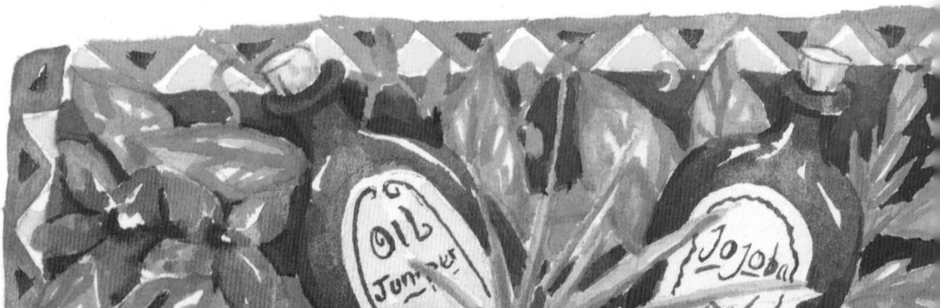

FOOT MASSAGE OIL

Massage this restorative oil firmly into tired and weary feet after a bath or shower, or a foot-bath.

40 ml (1½ fl oz) almond oil
5 ml (⅙ fl oz) avocado oil
5 ml (⅙ fl oz) wheatgerm oil
25 drops lime flower oil

CALENDULA MASSAGE OIL

Massage this oil liberally into your feet after bathing if you suffer from persistent soreness.

30 ml (1 fl oz) almond oil
15 ml (½ fl oz) avocado oil
5 ml (⅙ fl oz) wheatgerm oil
75 drops calendula oil

SWEATY FEET

First bathe feet in a bowl of hot water containing a few drops of lemongrass oil, then apply the following oil rub.

30 ml (1 fl oz) soya oil
18 drops lemongrass oil

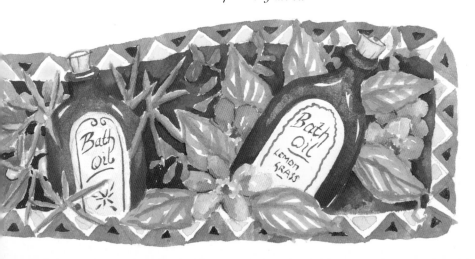

ATHLETICS, RUNNING, WALKING AND DANCING

When feet suffer from the rigours of demanding sports activity, soothe them with this healing massage oil.

25 ml (1 fl oz) almond oil
20 ml (⅔ fl oz) avocado oil
5 ml (⅙ fl oz) wheatgerm oil
20 drops rosemary oil
12 drops peppermint oil
16 drops lavender oil

FALLEN ARCHES

If the arches of your feet continually ache and cause pain, soak them in a therapeutic foot-bath, dry them, then massage each instep towards the heel of each foot with this soothing and comforting massage oil.

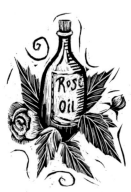

35 ml (1 fl oz) almond oil
20 ml (⅔ fl oz) avocado oil
5 ml (⅙ fl oz) wheatgerm oil
20 drops rosemary oil
10 drops black pepper oil
20 drops ginger oil
10 drops clary sage oil

Facial Oil Blends

Choose from the following facial massage oils to suit your particular skin type.

NORMAL SKIN

45 ml (1½ fl oz) hazelnut oil
5 ml (⅙ fl oz) jojoba oil
6 drops frankincense oil
6 drops geranium oil
3 drops jasmine oil
12 drops lavender oil

DRY SKIN

45 ml (1½ fl oz) hazelnut oil
5 ml (⅙ fl oz) jojoba oil
8 drops rose oil
8 drops chamomile oil
8 drops sandalwood oil

OILY SKIN

45 ml (1½ fl oz) hazelnut oil
5 ml (⅙ fl oz) jojoba oil
8 drops cedarwood oil
10 drops lemon oil
6 drops ylang-ylang oil

DID YOU KNOW . . . ?

That rose oil is the most valuable and useful of the natural perfumed oils, and that it takes approximately 30 roses to make just 1 drop of oil?

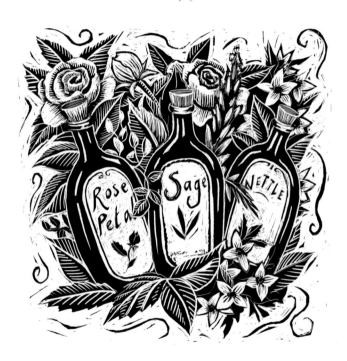

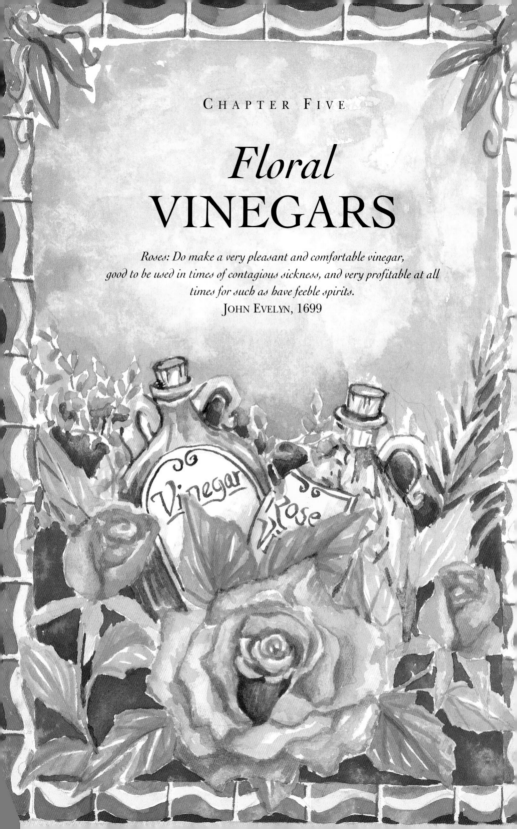

CHAPTER FIVE

Floral
VINEGARS

*Roses: Do make a very pleasant and comfortable vinegar,
good to be used in times of contagious sickness, and very profitable at all
times for such as have feeble spirits.*
JOHN EVELYN, 1699

Fragrant vinegars have been used for centuries to ward off infections, and as bath additives and beauty tonics. They are an easy way of making a bath delightfully aromatic, as well as softening the water and so helping to leave your skin feeling lovely and fresh.

Used regularly in dry climates — especially during winter — bath vinegars will keep your skin from drying and flaking. They can also be used as the basis of a natural deodorant or a facial toning lotion, and they have a far more refreshing scent than floral waters made with alcohol. When used in cooling compresses for the brow, floral vinegars can ease headaches and tension. Dab a little behind your ears and on your temples to relieve any fatigue or tension resulting from exposure to a hot sun.

Preparation of Floral Vinegars

Vinegars can be made from any fragrant herb or flower, singly or in combination, by following the directions in Chapter One. Herb seeds will also yield their beneficial properties to vinegars. They should be prepared by bruising the seeds with a pestle and mortar and allowing 2 teaspoons of seeds to every 1 litre (32 fl oz) of vinegar. Then add required amount to the recipe.

Fresh or Dried Herbs

Whenever possible, use fresh herbs or flower petals to make your vinegars. In most cases, the volatile essences will be at their optimum level when the plant is fresh.

Gather herbs in the early morning, when they are dry and before the sun has had a chance to draw out and disperse their volatile oil. Do not pick them if they are wet from rain or still damp with dew. Only collect sufficient for your immediate needs, and handle them as little as possible — herbs bruise easily. Avoid cross-flavouring by keeping different herbs separate and, as you pick them, lay the herbs out thinly on trays.

When gathering herbs it is also important to know what and when to harvest.

Flowers

Select only those which are unblemished and pick them when they are fully open.

Leaves

Volatile oils are at their peak just before the herb or plant flowers, and leaves should be picked then.

Seeds

Cut whole heads once they are brown and the seeds are ready to fall.

If you find it more convenient to use dried herbs, use only those that are no more than 12 months old and which have been stored in airtight containers or packages.

The procedure for preparing vinegars from dried herbs or petals is slightly different from that used with fresh plants. However, if you follow the directions in Chapter One you will still obtain an acceptable vinegar that will suit your needs.

Using Your Vinegars

In the Bath

Vinegars are more astringent than bath oils and are therefore particularly suitable for greasy skins.

Add 1 cup (250 ml/8 fl oz) of vinegar to the bath while the taps are running. Also, soak a soft face cloth in the vinegar, wring it out and lay it across your forehead while you lie back and relax in your bath.

BATH INVIGORATOR
500 ml (16 fl oz) cider vinegar
1 piece fresh ginger root, minced
4 sprigs rosemary
2 handfuls sage

Prepare vinegar as directed in Chapter One, and bottle for future use. Use in the bath to soothe tired muscles; it can also be dabbed onto problem areas such as spots with cottonwool.

Facial Toners

Unlike skin tonics made by the herbal infusion method, a vinegar-based facial toner will last indefinitely.

When you cleanse facial skin, pores are opened slightly. It is therefore important to use an astringent to close them again, firming the skin at the same time. Toners will also remove the last traces of grease, dead cells, grime and soap, as well as helping to redress the skin's pH balance.

DRY SKIN	*Rose petals and elder flowers are gentle and soothing. Lime flowers (linden blossom) will help to smooth out wrinkles.*
NORMAL SKIN	*Good herbs to use are marigold, meadowsweet, marshmallow, elder flower and rose. For a slightly more astringent effect, combine rose and witch-hazel.*
OILY SKIN	*Use yarrow, sage, rosemary and horsetail (Equisetum arvense). For extremely oily skin with over-large pores, use a combination of equal parts of sage, yarrow and witch-hazel. Its antiseptic properties are also helpful if you get an occasional outbreak of spots.*
SENSITIVE SKIN	*Choose from elder flower, marigold, rose petals and chamomile. These herbs can be used singly or in combination. For extra astringency, include witch-hazel.*
COMBINATION SKIN	*Use a slightly astringent toner for the oily panels. For the rest of the face, choose a gentle toner from those recommended for normal or dry skin.*

Prepare your herbal vinegar as directed in Chapter One, then dilute it — 20 ml (⅔ fl oz) of vinegar to every 150 ml (5 fl oz) of distilled water. Bottle and store it in an airtight container with a non-metallic lid.

Pour a little toner onto slightly damp cottonwool and gently apply to face and neck, using an outward and upward movement.

FACE WASH

2 tablespoons lavender vinegar
1 cup (250 ml/8 fl oz) rose-water

Mix vinegar and rose-water thoroughly and store in a tightly-capped bottle. Apply directly to the face.

It is very simple to create an astringent vinegar face wash to suit your individual needs. Choose from any of the herbs for Fragrant Washing Waters in Chapter One, either alone or mixed, and dilute the herbal vinegar with distilled water.

Other herbs and flowers to include are:

BASIL • DILL • SWEET-SCENTED GERANIUM LEAVES • HONEYSUCKLE
JASMINE • LEMON VERBENA • VIOLET

HEADACHE

125 ml (4 fl oz) lavender vinegar
250 ml (8 fl oz) rose-water

Blend the ingredients well and store in a tightly-sealed bottle. Whenever headache from stress or strain persists, lay a handkerchief dampened with vinegar across your forehead for 5–10 minutes. Try this in a relaxing bath.

Sun Exposure

After exposure to a hot sun, dab lavender, rose or lemon verbena vinegar behind your ears and to your temples and forehead.

Vinaigrettes

Vinaigrettes, or 'smelling bottles', are small glass bottles containing a piece of sponge and fragrant vinegar. Their popularity peaked in the Regency period, when people carried them to allay the fetid odours prevalent in crowded places. Today, these delightful 'smelling bottles' make a useful addition to the bathroom cabinet or medicine chest. Hold them under your nose to relieve a stuffy head or headache, or to ward off any feelings of faintness.

COTTAGE GARDEN VINAIGRETTE

2 tablespoons dried rose petals
2 tablespoons dried lavender
1 tablespoon dried rosemary
1 tablespoon dried marjoram
5 ml (⅙ fl oz) camphorated oil (from the chemist)
200 ml (6½ fl oz) white wine vinegar

Put the herbs into a wide-mouthed glass jar. Gently warm the vinegar and pour into the jar. Seal the jar tightly and leave it where it will receive plenty of sun for 2 weeks. Shake the contents every day.

Strain the vinegar and mix in the camphorated oil. Push a small piece of natural sponge into a suitable bottle, add the vinegar and seal tightly.

To use, remove the lid from the bottle, hold it under your nose and breathe deeply to freshen and clear your head.

DID YOU KNOW . . . ?

That for many centuries aromatic vinegars were thought to ward off infections, and that in Regency England little bottles of moss soaked in vinegar were carried by fashionable young people wherever they went.

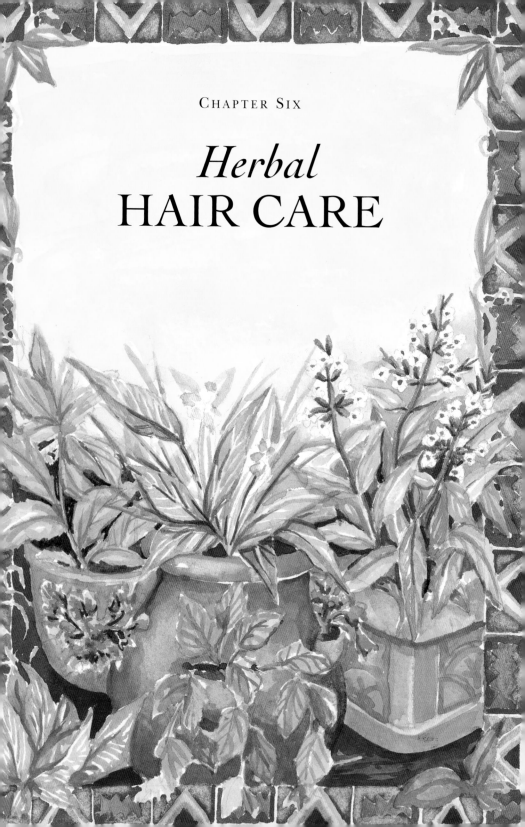

CHAPTER SIX

Herbal
HAIR CARE

Herbs for Beautiful Hair

Beautifully clean, bouncy, shiny hair is without doubt an enviable asset. To maintain your hair's good looks you must also maintain all-round good health, for the condition of your hair is usually a good indication of the state of your general health. If you feel even slightly out-of-sorts, it is surprising how quickly your hair will lose its sheen and body. Maintaining a healthy, balanced diet is essential, for your hair needs vitamin B complex, vitamin A, calcium, silica, iron, zinc, protein and unsaturated oils or fatty acids. Eat plenty of fresh fruit, vegetables and salads, drink lots of water and make sure that you get enough sleep — eight hours' rest each night will do wonders for your hair.

Although diet is the foundation of healthy hair, herbs will also help to bring out its natural beauty. Their gentle cleansing and conditioning action will leave hair shiny and manageable, ensuring that healthy lustre and bounce that everyone notices. Those old-fashioned tips from grandma's day, like shampooing with an egg to bring life to dry hair, and using a lemon juice or vinegar rinse for oily hair, still work. Similarly, traditional herbal rinses made from rosemary, nettle or yarrow massaged into the scalp after shampooing will stimulate hair growth and help control dandruff and over-active sebaceous glands.

You are not quite like anyone else and your hair is not quite like anyone else's hair, either. What better way to cater for your hair's needs than to use a 'personalised' natural shampoo! Unlike their commercial counterparts, shampoos made at home contain no synthetics, detergents or chemicals, in particular, no environmentally-damaging phosphates. They may not produce mountains of froth like the store-bought varieties, but they will leave your hair feeling squeaky clean and healthy.

Normal Hair

Normal hair has well-balanced sebaceous glands which provide just the right amount of sebum to lubricate each hair shaft. This type of hair normally looks clean, and the ends are resistant to splitting.

Dry Hair

This very common hair type benefits from external treatments such as herbal conditioning oils, as well as from a diet that includes beneficial foods such as protein, cereals, nuts, fish, lean meat, fresh fruit and vegetables.

So-called 'beauty treatments' and fashion trends such as bleaching, dying, harsh perms, heated rollers, tongs and back combing should be avoided, as they can have a devastating effect on dry hair.

Oily Hair

People with oily hair need to exercise patience in its treatment so that a correct balance is found. Quite often too much washing will actually make the condition worse because it overstimulates the sebaceous glands. However, not washing your hair at all can also create a problem, leaving you with an unsightly mess of lank, stringy hair.

Washing hair as often as required with an appropriate gentle herbal shampoo will help correct over-active sebaceous glands. Herbs such as rosemary, lavender, lemon and yarrow are excellent for this purpose.

Pre-Wash Conditioning

As with the rest of your skin, your scalp can be affected by dry climatic conditions, leaving you with a flaky scalp or dandruff. This condition can be remedied with regular use of a mildly antiseptic pre-wash conditioner that will stimulate, cleanse and moisturise your scalp.

This conditioner has an almond oil base which is similar to your own scalp oil, acting as an excellent emollient to protect your skin and replace natural surface oils, preventing roughness and chapping. Certain herbs have also been included for their therapeutic benefits: peppermint for its cleansing effect on the scalp and its mildly antiseptic, stimulating and aromatic qualities, rosemary as an effective control against dandruff, and fennel for its healing properties.

CONDITIONER
200 ml (6½ fl oz) almond oil
2 teaspoons dried peppermint
2 teaspoons dried rosemary
1 teaspoon fennel seed

Fill a suitable wide-mouthed glass jar with the almond oil, then add the herbs. Seal the jar tightly and place it where it will receive plenty of hot sunlight for at least 14 days. Strain and repeat the procedure with a fresh batch of herbs. Carefully strain the herb oil and store in an airtight amber-coloured glass bottle.

Massage a little oil into your scalp whenever it needs extra conditioning, or when dry and flaky skin is evident.

FOR HAIR THAT TANGLES

For dry hair that tangles when wet, pre-condition with a few drops of a blend of equal parts of rosemary oil and lavender oil. Massage well into your scalp about half an hour before shampooing.

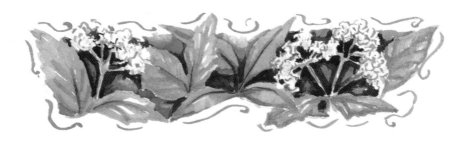

PROTEIN CONDITIONER FOR DAMAGED HAIR

Brittle, damaged hair can be given strength and lustre by being treated with this rich protein conditioner.

60 ml (2 fl oz) castor oil
3 tablespoons anhydrous lanolin
40 ml (1½ fl oz) almond oil
80 ml (3 fl oz) glycerine
20 ml (⅔ fl oz) baby shampoo
1¼ cups (310 ml/10 fl oz) warm water
2 eggs
2 egg yolks
10 ml (⅓ fl oz) cider vinegar
few drops rosemary oil

Put the lanolin, castor and almond oils in a double saucepan and melt together over medium heat. When completely liquid, remove from the heat and allow to stand for 5 minutes. Using an electric beater, whisk in the glycerine, baby shampoo and water. As the mixture thickens, add the egg yolks, cider vinegar and then the rosemary oil, a drop at a time, until the mixture is sufficiently scented. Pour into a sterilised glass jar with a tight-fitting lid, and refrigerate for 24 hours.

To use, beat 2 eggs at high speed and add to mixture, then massage into newly shampooed hair. Cover with a shower cap and leave on for at least one hour, then shampoo out with *Fragile Hair Shampoo* (see page 92). Finish by rinsing several times with *Rosemary Conditioning Rinse.*

Apply this conditioning treatment weekly until your hair has regained its strength and lustre, then reduce treatment to once a month.

PROTEIN CONDITIONER

This is a quick and easy weekly treatment to nourish your hair and keep it looking shiny and healthy.

20 ml (²⁄₃ fl oz) almond oil
20 ml (²⁄₃ fl oz) wheatgerm oil
20 ml (²⁄₃ fl oz) glycerine
10 ml (¹⁄₃ fl oz) cider vinegar
3 drops rosemary oil
3 drops carrot oil
2 eggs

Put all the ingredients in a ceramic bowl and beat vigorously until thoroughly mixed. After shampooing, apply the mixture, working it well into the hair, then cover with a shower cap. Leave for 20 minutes, then shampoo out using lukewarm water (so as not to scramble the egg!). To finish, use a herbal conditioning rinse appropriate to your hair type.

Shampoos

Herbs and essential oils can be added to a shampoo base to clean various hair types and to treat different conditions that affect the hair and scalp.

Make your shampoo base by whichever method you find most convenient.

SOAPWORT SHAMPOO

This is made from the dried roots of the soapwort plant (*Saponaria officinalis*). This herb has natural cleansing qualities. It contains a mildly foaming substance called saponin which makes it ideal to use as a shampoo base.

Soapwort shampoo is especially effective for dry, permed, dyed or heat-damaged hair. It is also used for itchy scalp conditions such as dermatitis.

Dried soapwort root can be purchased from specialist herb suppliers, some health food stores and herbalists. Choose from any of the herbs listed under Shampoo Herbs (see page 84) and add them to the following recipe:

2 tablespoons dried soapwort root, chopped
1 tablespoon dried herb of choice
1 litre (32 fl oz) distilled water

Bring the soapwort root and distilled water to the boil in an enamel or stainless steel saucepan. Simmer for 20 minutes, keeping the saucepan covered. Remove from the heat, add your chosen herbs, cover, and infuse until cold. Strain through fine muslin, then drip through coffee filter paper. Store in an empty shampoo bottle. Use within 7 days.

ALMOND OIL SHAMPOO

This is an excellent moisturising shampoo base for scalp skin which has become dry and flaky.

10 ml (⅓ fl oz) almond oil
5 ml (⅙ fl oz) glycerine
5 drops carrot oil
1 cup (250 ml/8 fl oz) herbal infusion

Prepare the infusion from the list of Shampoo Herbs appropriate to your hair type and needs on page 84. Combine the ingredients in an old shampoo bottle, or other suitable container, and shake well until blended.

HERBAL SHAMPOO INFUSION

To prepare the infusion, put 2 to 3 teaspoonfuls of herbs, alone or in combination, in a ceramic bowl and add 625 ml (20 fl oz) of boiling water. Cover and steep until cold, then strain through muslin, drip through coffee filter paper and add required amount to shampoo base recipe.

Any leftover infusion can be added to your bathwater.

SOAP BASE SHAMPOO

An excellent shampoo to make when you need enough for all the family.

Use only pure soap or soap flakes for this convenient, long-lasting shampoo.

2 litres (64 fl oz) distilled water
100 g (3½ fl oz) soap flakes, or finely-grated soap
juice of ½ lemon (optional)

Bring the water to the boil, then reduce to a simmer and add the soap flakes or grated soap. Return mixture to the boil and stir continuously until the soap has dissolved. Remove from heat, add the lemon juice and stir until well mixed. Let the mixture cool, then bottle it in a wide-mouthed jar or similar container. The lemon juice can be omitted in favour of essential oils, if you prefer. If substituting essential oils, add approximately 10 drops of the oils nominated under your hair type to each 100 ml (3½ fl oz) of this base.

The mixture will gel and may become lumpy when left for a while. Simply shake it vigorously or beat it up in a blender.

DRY SHAMPOO

A busy schedule can make it impossible to wash your hair when it needs it the most. This is when a dry shampoo is the answer — in 10 minutes your hair will be clean and looking good again.

15 g (½ oz) fuller's earth
15 g (½ oz) orris root powder
15 g (½ oz) arrowroot
10 drops rosemary oil

Fuller's earth is available from the chemist and usually comes in powdered form. (If it is not, reduce it to a powder using a mortar and pestle.) Mix the rest of the ingredients in with the fuller's earth, and then pass the powder through a fine sieve. Store in an airtight container.

To use, sprinkle a small amount over your hair and gently massage in with your fingers. Leave it for 10 minutes, then brush it out using a soft-bristled brush.

INSTANT HERBAL SHAMPOO

This shampoo works very well in hard water and will last indefinitely. It is also a must for people who travel, as it is light and takes up almost no space.

1 tablespoon dried lavender
1 tablespoon dried yarrow
1 tablespoon dried lime flowers, or other fragrant herb
1 tablespoon dried chamomile for blonde hair, or dried rosemary for dark hair
1 tablespoon baking soda
2 tablespoons pure, grated soap

Finely grind all herbs with a mortar and pestle and mix them with the soap flakes and baking soda. Store in an airtight container.

Mix a teaspoon of the dry shampoo with a small quantity of water and massage well into your scalp and hair, then rinse.

PROTEIN SHAMPOO FOR DRY HAIR

Use this shampoo twice a week to cleanse and bring life to dry hair.

Whisk one egg white. Massage this through dry hair. Leave it on for at least five minutes. Add the lightly beaten egg yolk and gently massage it into hair and scalp. Rinse out with lukewarm water — under no circumstances use hot water, or you will scramble the egg!

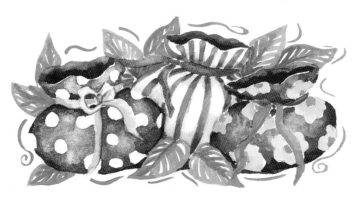

Shampoo Herbs

Choose from any of the following herbs and make a personalised shampoo to suit your particular hair type. Use the herbs singly or in combinations.

HERB	PROPERTIES	HAIR TYPE
CHAMOMILE	Anti-inflammatory and healing for scalp irritations. Acts as a tonic for fair hair and has a lightening effect, giving yellow highlights.	Dry, Normal, or Fair
COMFREY	Healing herb for irritated scalp conditions. Make an infusion from the leaf or a decoction from the root.	Dry
ELDER FLOWERS	A gentle hair stimulant. Anti-inflammatory and healing for the scalp.	All types

LEMON BALM	Gentle cleansing action. Imparts a delightful lemony scent to the hair.	Oily
LEMONGRASS	Lemon-scented cleansing herb.	Oily
LEMON VERBENA	Cleansing herb and pore stimulant.	All types
MARSHMALLOW	Has a softening and conditioning effect.	Dry
NETTLE	Stimulating to the circulation of the scalp; helps cleanse the hair gently.	All types
PARSLEY	Healing for scalp conditions and stimulating for the hair. Balances the sebaceous glands.	All types
PEPPERMINT	Has a purifying effect on the scalp. Mildly antiseptic, stimulating and aromatic.	All types
RED CLOVER	Gentle cleansing herb.	Dry
ROSEMARY	Helps control dandruff. Brings out the highlights of deeper shades of hair colour.	All types, Dark
SAGE	Helps close the pores of the skin. Enhances darker colour tones.	Normal, or Oily

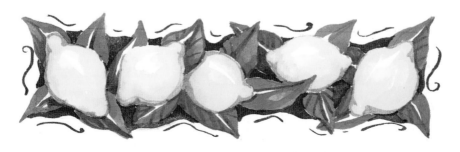

SOUTHERNWOOD	Cleansing, antiseptic herb that keeps the scalp healthy and stimulates the hair follicles. It has a pungent scent, so it is best combined with an aromatic herb such as lavender. Prepare as a decoction, see Chapter One.	All types
THYME	Cleansing and tonic herb. Has anti-dandruff properties. Imparts a beautiful fresh fragrance to the hair.	All types
YARROW	Refreshing and cleansing, acts as a tonic for the hair. Helps control over-active sebaceous glands.	Oily

Shampoo Oils

Like herbs, essential oils help improve the general health of your hair and scalp, and can also be used to control various conditions such as dandruff. They are best added to the *Soap Base Shampoo*, alone or in combination. Since they are very potent, you should add no more than 10 to 12 drops in total, unless otherwise directed.

Essential oils to use are:

NORMAL	DRY	OILY	FRAGILE	DANDRUFF
lavender	lavender	lavender	lavender	lavender
rosemary	rosemary	rosemary	calendula	rosemary
lemon	geranium	cypress	parsley	lemon
parsley	carrot	lemon	chamomile	thyme
geranium	parsley	basil	thyme	basil
carrot	yarrow	sage	carrot	cypress
	sandalwood	thyme	sandalwood	sage
		clary sage		

Looking After Your Hair

Our hair is made of a substance called keratin, which is basically the same material that fingernails are made from. Although the hair we see is technically dead, it still mirrors to a great extent what is happening inside and outside our bodies.

Hair is kept healthy by maintaining a balanced diet and doing adequate exercise. If you eat plenty of fresh food, cut down on stimulants such as coffee, tea and alcohol, increase your vitamin B dosage, use only cold-pressed oils and unsaturated fatty acids and make sure that you get enough sleep, you will end up with beautiful, shiny hair.

What most people put on their hair is usually an unknown chemical cocktail that may have dubious results. Taking a natural approach — using non-detergent based shampoos with your own blend of herbs or oils — will guarantee that your hair and scalp remain healthy. Natural products are also less likely to strip your hair of its protective acid mantle.

Choose from those herbs and essential oils recommended for your hair type, combining them to suit your particular needs, or simply use the following recipes. Observing these basic rules will help you get the best results:

* *When you wash your hair, have the water comfortably warm. Very cold or very hot water are both too much of a shock to the scalp.*

* *Wet your hair thoroughly before applying shampoo.*

* *Use shampoo sparingly.*

* *Wash your hair only when necessary; washing too frequently can overstimulate the scalp and leave your hair with dry, brittle ends.*

* *Rinse out all traces of shampoo and conditioner before drying your hair. Rinse until the water runs clear — a shower attachment makes this easier.*

* *Pat the hair dry with a towel. Do not rub the hair or scalp hard. If possible, sit back in the sun and relax while you gently flick the moisture out with your fingertips, or loosely wrap it in a towel and let it dry naturally.*

* *Do not brush wet hair — you will split the ends and pull it out by the roots.*

* *Use a very wide-toothed comb to gently comb out your hair.*

* *It is best to avoid curling tongs, heated rollers and hair driers — excessive use wil' dry hair and make it brittle. Never use a hair drier on dripping wet hair. If you must use one, towel your hair dry first and then use the drier on a warm or cool setting.*

* *Do not brush hair excessively or tease it, both will aggravate brittle and oily hair conditions. If you must tease your hair, do it in sections, starting at the roots.*

* *Use a pre-wash conditioner before shampooing to take care of dry ends.*

※ *Do not use elastic bands on your hair — they can cause hair to split. Use a covered band instead.*

※ *Do not pull hair back tightly into a bun or ponytail. This will break your hair and cause it to split.*

※ *Avoid using chemical bleaches and dyes — they may cause skin irritations and even dermatitis, in some people. There are safe and effective herbal alternatives.*

※ *Before styling, dampen your hair by using a pump-spray filled with water or herbal setting lotion. It will direct a controlled fine spray.*

※ *Always keep brushes and combs scrupulously clean. Wash them in a diluted rosemary decoction (see Decoction, Chapter One) to eliminate grease buildup.*

※ *Have your hair cut about every six weeks to keep the style in shape and get rid of split ends.*

※ *After swimming in salt or chlorinated water, wash your hair with a herbal shampoo and then rinse with a conditioner. Apply a conditioner to your hair before you go swimming. As you swim it will slowly rinse away, protecting your hair from the harshness of chlorine or salt water.*

Normal Hair

A good shampoo for normal hair can be made by adding an infusion made from the following herbs to either the *Almond Oil Shampoo* (see page 82) or the *Soap Base Shampoo* (see page 82).

FAIR HAIR
2 tablespoons dried chamomile
2 tablespoons dried yarrow
1 tablespoon dried lime flowers
2 teaspoons dried fennel seeds
2 litres (64 fl oz) boiling water

DARK HAIR
2 tablespoons dried sage
2 tablespoons dried rosemary
1 tablespoon dried lime flowers
2 teaspoons dried fennel seed
2 litres (64 fl oz) boiling water

Prepare the infusion as directed in Chapter One and add required amount directed in the recipe of your choice.

MONTHLY CLEANSING TREATMENT

The following cleansing treatment can be used once a month in conjunction with your other shampoo to both clean the hair and scalp and replace natural oils lost through shampooing.

30 ml (1 fl oz) almond oil
30 ml (1 fl oz) castor oil
185 ml (6 fl oz) herbal infusion

Prepare the herbal infusion as previously directed (see Chapter One), using 4 tablespoons of dried herb to 1 litre (32 fl oz) of boiling water. Use chamomile for fair hair and rosemary for dark hair.

MOISTURISING SHAMPOO

This shampoo is made by adding essential oils to the *Soap Base Shampoo* (see page 82).

200 ml (6½ fl oz) Soap Base Shampoo *(see page 82)*
6 drops geranium oil
8 drops carrot oil
4 drops lemon oil
8 drops rosemary oil

Mix all ingredients thoroughly in a blender, and store in an old shampoo bottle or other suitable container. Shake well before use, as the mixture may gel.

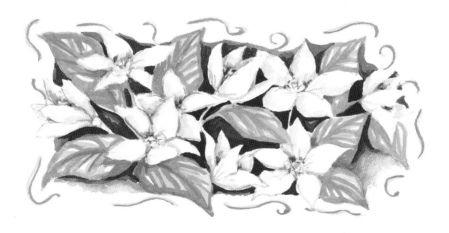

Dry Hair

S H A M P O O

To the *Soap Base Shampoo* (see page 82), add an infusion of the following herbs:

2 tablespoons dried chamomile
2 tablespoons dried elder flowers
2 litres (64 fl oz) boiling water
1 tablespoon marshmallow
1 tablespoon parsley

Prepare the infusion (see Chapter One) and add required amount as directed in the base recipe.

M O I S T U R I S I N G   S H A M P O O

Add the following essential oils to the *Soap Base Shampoo* (see page 82):

200 ml (6½ fl oz) Soap Base Shampoo (see page 82)
10 ml (⅓ fl oz) almond oil
2 ml (¹⁄₁₂ fl oz) jojoba oil
5 drops carrot oil
2 drops rosemary oil

S C A L P   M A S S A G E

A scalp massage will help keep dry hair in better condition. Each evening before going to bed, press your fingertips against your scalp and rotate the scalp underneath them gently.

Oily Hair

S H A M P O O

The best approach for this type of hair is to wash it as often as required with any of the shampoo bases, plus appropriate herbs or essential oils. *Soapwort Shampoo* is excellent for treating this type of hair condition.

2 tablespoons dried lavender
2 tablespoons dried lemon balm
2 litres (64 fl oz) boiling water
1 tablespoon dried rosemary
1 tablespoon dried yarrow

Prepare infusion as directed in Chapter One, then add 2 to 3 tablespoons to the *Soapwort Shampoo* recipe (see page 81).

STIMULATING SHAMPOO

200 ml (6½ fl oz) Soap Base Shampoo *(see page 82)*
6 drops rosemary oil
4 drops lavender oil
20 drops lemon oil
4 drops cypress oil

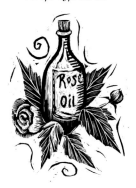

DRY SHAMPOO FOR OILY HAIR

45 g (1½ g) fuller's earth
8 drops lemon oil
4 drops rosemary oil

Prepare as directed for *Dry Shampoo*, see page 83.

Sprinkle a small amount over your hair and massage in well with your fingertips. After 10 minutes, brush out with a soft-bristled brush.

After Shampoo Care

Be gentle when drying — 'mop' out excess water and wrap your hair in a towel to help it dry. Do not drag the bristles of the brush across your scalp when you brush; let your hair fall forward and brush gently, so that the oils are taken to the ends of the hair.

Diet also plays an important part in looking after and controlling oily hair. Eat plenty of fresh fruit and vegetables, drink at least 8 glasses of water a day to keep your body cleansed, and drink herbal teas, such as yarrow.

Fragile and Damaged Hair

This condition usually results from too many perms, bleaching, colouring, mousses and gels, all of which result in hair that is thin, split or breaks on touching.

To help correct the problem, the scalp needs to be stimulated to encourage new and stronger growth. Until the new hair is at the length that you want it, the fragile hair needs to be treated with great care and washed with an appropriate shampoo.

You may find it necessary to use more than one of these recommended shampoo recipes. Add the following herbal infusions to either of the shampoo bases (*Soapwort Shampoo*, see page 81, *Soap Base Shampoo*, see page 82) in the quantities directed:

DAMAGED HAIR SHAMPOO
2 tablespoons dried chamomile
2 tablespoons dried rosemary
2 tablespoons dried peppermint
1 tablespoon dried borage flowers
1 litre (32 fl oz) boiling water

As well as using this shampoo, you should also treat your hair with the *Protein Conditioner for Damaged Hair*, see page 80.

STIMULATING SHAMPOO
200 ml (6½ fl oz) Soap Base Shampoo *(see page 82)*
4 drops lavender oil
4 drops parsley seed oil

Blend all ingredients thoroughly. Use once a week.

CONDITIONING SHAMPOO
200 ml (6½ fl oz) Soap Base Shampoo (see page 82)
5 ml (⅙ fl oz) jojoba oil
6 drops chamomile oil
4 drops lavender oil

Blend all ingredients thoroughly. Use in place of regular shampoo until hair begins to regain its natural condition.

TO PROMOTE HAIR GROWTH
1 tablespoon dried rosemary
2 tablespoons dried southernwood
1 tablespoon dried yarrow
625 ml (20 fl oz) boiling water

Prepare the infusion as directed, and store in an airtight bottle in the refrigerator for up to 7 days.

Massage into scalp morning and night.

TO THICKEN HAIR
Apply this treatment to the scalp and hair once a month.

250 ml (8 fl oz) clear honey
200 ml (6½ fl oz) almond oil
50 ml (2 fl oz) hazelnut oil
250 ml (8 fl oz) herbal infusion

Prepare the herbal infusion as directed in Chapter One, using chamomile for fair hair and rosemary for dark hair.

Blend all the ingredients thoroughly, then rub the mixture well into the hair and scalp. Cover with a plastic shower cap and leave on for half an hour. Shampoo out using one of the *Fragile Hair Shampoos* (see page 92). Any leftover mixture can be kept in the refrigerator for the next treatment.

Falling Hair

This can result from an illness or becoming run down, or be due to a major hormonal upset. We all shed hair every day of our lives, and whenever you comb or brush there will be hair loss. However, when you start to notice that more hair is coming away in your hairbrush than normal, then it is time to treat your falling hair.

This condition is not as serious as hair loss and you may find that a course of brewer's yeast tablets will help. Also, check your diet — include plenty of fresh fruit and vegetables, cut down on stimulants such as coffee, tea and alcohol, and drink plenty of fresh water. Check your haircare habits, making sure that you are not using hair dryers excessively.

Use any of the shampoos which are applicable to your hair type, and add a beaten egg to a small amount of the mixture each time you wash your hair. Do not use hot water or the egg will scramble. Leave it on for as long as possible — at least a few minutes, if you are under the shower or in the bath — before rinsing out.

Include a weekly treatment of the *Protein Conditioner*, see page 81. After shampooing, use the appropriate hair conditioner and final rinse for *Falling Hair* (see page 100).

CONDITIONING SHAMPOO
200 ml (6½ fl oz) Soap Base Shampoo *(see page 82)*
5 ml (⅛ fl oz) jojoba oil
6 drops rosemary oil
4 drops chamomile oil

Prepare *Soap Base Shampoo* as directed on page 82, then add essential oils and mix thoroughly.

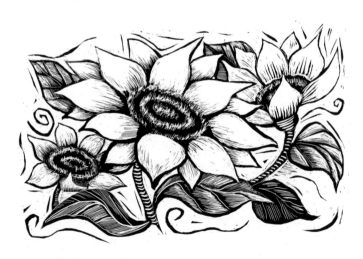

Herbal Conditioners and Rinses

A natural conditioner gives added health and shine to your hair. If you use it two or three times a week it will help replace scalp oil lost through washing, remove any remaining shampoo residue, and balance the scalp's pH levels.

There are many different ways you can use the beneficial properties of herbs for conditioning hair. The simplest is probably to make a base from lecithin, a protein extracted from soya beans. Lecithin is available in granule and liquid form from health food stores. The thick orange liquid makes a superb conditioning base.

CONDITIONING BASE

100 ml (3½ fl oz) liquid lecithin
75 ml (2½ fl oz) almond oil
25 ml (1 fl oz) peach kernel oil
20 ml (⅔ fl oz) jojoba oil
10 g (⅓ oz) cocoa butter

Put the cocoa butter in a double saucepan and melt over medium heat. When completely liquefied, add the remaining ingredients and stir until melted and blended. Remove from the heat and pour into a sterilised wide-mouthed glass jar.

Use as directed, according to hair type.

CONDITIONING RINSE

To make a conditioning rinse, place the appropriate herbs for your hair type in a ceramic bowl and pour boiling water over them. Steep overnight, strain through muslin and add lemon juice or cider vinegar, as directed. Store in a tightly-sealed bottle in the refrigerator for up to 7 days.

After washing and conditioning your hair, rinse thoroughly with clean water and finish by pouring the herbal rinse through. Repeat several times, each time rubbing rinse well into your hair.

ROSEMARY HAIR LOTION

This after-shampoo conditioning lotion is suitable for all hair types. It will help revitalise the scalp and hair and will also help prevent dandruff. For more specific needs, use one of the Rinses listed under your particular hair type.

Put 6 fresh, leafy rosemary stalks in an enamel saucepan, add 5 cups (1.25 litres/2 pints) of distilled water and bring to the boil. Reduce heat and simmer for 30 minutes, keeping the lid on so that the vapour does not escape. Remove from the heat, steep until cold and strain through fine muslin.

Use as final rinse after thoroughly rinsing out all traces of shampoo and conditioner. Massage well into your scalp with your fingertips.

Normal Hair

MOISTURISING CONDITIONER

40 ml (1½ fl oz) Conditioning Base *(see page 95)*
45 ml (1½ fl oz) hazelnut oil
5 ml (⅛ fl oz) wheatgerm oil
6 drops carrot oil
4 drops rosemary oil

Thoroughly blend all ingredients in a double saucepan over medium heat. When cool, apply all over the hair, massaging through with your fingers. Leave on for 5 to 10 minutes before rinsing out.

HERBAL RINSE

FAIR HAIR	DARK HAIR
1 tablespoon dried chamomile	*1 tablespoon dried rosemary*
2 teaspoons dried elder flowers	*2 teaspoons dried elder flowers*
2 teaspoons dried nettles	*2 teaspoons dried nettles*
2 litres (64 fl oz) boiling water	*2 litres (64 fl oz) boiling water*

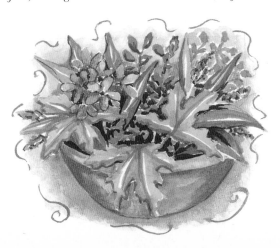

pH RINSE

1 tablespoon lemon juice
1¼ litres (40 fl oz) water
3 drops lemon oil

Mix all ingredients in an airtight glass bottle, shaking well before use.

Once a week, after shampooing, use this as your final rinse to restore the natural pH balance of your hair.

Dry Hair

NOURISHING CONDITIONER

10 ml (⅓ fl oz) Conditioning Base (see page 95)
10 ml (⅓ fl oz) sesame oil
40 ml (1½ fl oz) sunflower oil
40 ml (1½ fl oz) hazelnut oil
6 drops rosemary oil
4 drops carrot oil
4 drops evening primrose oil
8 drops geranium oil

Prepare as for *Moisturising Conditioner*. Apply to the scalp and hair while the mixture is still warm but not hot, and massage in well with your fingers. Rinse out after 5 to 10 minutes with clean water. For a final rinse, pour through the *Rosemary Hair Lotion* (see page 95).

HERBAL RINSE FOR SUN-DAMAGED HAIR

2 tablespoons dried chamomile
2 tablespoons dried rosemary
2 tablespoons dried peppermint
1 tablespoon dried marshmallow
2 litres (64 fl oz) boiling water

Prepare a herbal infusion as directed in Chapter One. Use as a final rinse, massaging well into the hair and scalp with your fingertips.

pH RINSE

1 tablespoon cider vinegar
1¼ litres (40 fl oz) water
3 drops sandalwood oil

Thoroughly mix all ingredients in an airtight glass bottle, shaking well before use.

Once a week, after shampooing, use this as your final rinse to restore the pH balance of your hair.

RESTORING LOTION FOR DULL HAIR

Brush a little of this lotion into your hair after shampooing to restore its shine and lustre.

6 teaspoons dried rosemary
2 teaspoons dried chamomile
510 ml (10 fl oz) boiling water
15 ml (½ fl oz) almond oil
5 ml (⅙ fl oz) peach kernel oil
4 drops rosemary oil

Prepare the herbal infusion as directed in Chapter One, steeping dried rosemary and dried chamomile in boiling water.

Blend oils with 250 ml (8 fl oz) of the herbal infusion in an airtight glass bottle, shaking well to mix.

Oily Hair

CONTROL CONDITIONER

40 ml (1½ fl oz) Conditioning Base (see page 95)
10 ml (⅓ fl oz) sesame seed oil
10 ml (⅓ fl oz) rum
20 ml (⅔ fl oz) yarrow infusion
6 drops rosemary oil
6 drops lavender oil
4 drops yarrow oil
2 eggs, separated
juice of half a lemon

Prepare the infusion as directed in Chapter One, using 3 teaspoonfuls of dried herb to 250 ml (8 fl oz) of boiling water. Add required amount to recipe.

Put the *Conditioning Base* in a double saucepan and melt over medium heat. When completely liquefied, add the sesame oil, rum and yarrow infusion, stirring continually until well blended. Remove mixture from heat, pour into a ceramic bowl and allow to cool. Add the essential oils and egg yolks, mixing thoroughly. Smear the mixture over your hair, working well in with your fingers. Leave on for 10 minutes.

To shampoo the *Control Conditioner* from your hair, beat the egg whites with the juice of half a lemon until stiff. Use this frothy mixture to wash your hair. Rinse your hair thoroughly and finish off with the *pH Conditioning Rinse*. This treatment will give your hair body, and a very healthy sheen.

pH CONDITIONING RINSE
2 teaspoons dried rosemary
2 teaspoons dried lavender
2 teaspoons dried yarrow
1¼ litres (40 fl oz) boiling water
1 tablespoon cider vinegar
3 drops rosemary oil

Infuse the herbs in the boiling water. Strain, then add the cider vinegar and rosemary oil to the liquid. Pour rinse through your hair several times after shampooing and rinsing clean. Massage through your hair and to the tips with your fingers.

RESTORING LUSTRE TO DULL HAIR
2 eggs
250 ml (8 fl oz) vodka
250 ml (8 fl oz) rose-water

Whisk eggs and vodka into the rose-water, then massage the mixture through your hair thoroughly, working it right out to the tips with your fingers. Leave on for 15 minutes, then rinse thoroughly with *Rosemary Lotion* (see page 95).

Fragile Hair
Use the *Protein Conditioner for Damaged Hair* (see page 80), as directed.

Falling Hair
Use the *Protein Conditioner* (see page 81), as directed.

NOURISHING CONDITIONER

20 ml (⅔ fl oz) Conditioning Base (see page 95)
30 ml (1 fl oz) hazelnut oil
30 ml (1 fl oz) almond oil
10 drops evening primrose oil
5 drops rosemary oil

Melt the *Conditioning Base,* hazelnut oil and almond oil together in a double saucepan over medium heat. When completely liquefied, remove from heat, allow to cool and stir in the essential oils.

Apply conditioner to hair, working in gently with the fingers. Leave on for 10 minutes before rinsing out. Finish with the following *pH Rinse,* massaging it gently through your hair.

pH RINSE

1 tablespoon cider vinegar
1¼ litres (40 fl oz) water
3 drops rosemary oil
3 drops lavender oil

Thoroughly blend all ingredients and apply after conditioning and rinsing your hair, massaging gently into the scalp and hair. Repeat several times to ensure good coverage and penetration.

Dandruff

Those telltale flakes of dead skin cells scattered on your shoulders are a good indication that your head and hair are in bad condition. Even if you brush your hair thoroughly in the morning and brush your shoulders before leaving the house, by the middle of the day those embarrassing white flakes are back again.

Food allergies and over-sugary diets can often promote dandruff. So watch your diet and try to see if there is any correlation between what you have eaten in the past 48 hours and how bad your scalp condition is. Cut down on excessively spicy foods, fat and sugar, very starchy white flour products and alcohol (particularly spirits) as far as possible. Eat plenty of raw vegetables and fruits, vegetable oils and nuts, lean meat and fish. Correct eating goes a long way towards improving this condition.

If you find that modification of your diet and the use of home-made herbal preparations do not work, and you are suffering scalp inflammation, bleeding or other severe irritation, you should immediately see a doctor, medical herbalist, dermatologist or trichologist.

Most cases of dandruff will respond well to home treatments, and combining the external applications with a good internal regime should give positive results quite quickly.

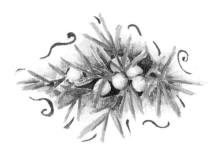

ANTI-DANDRUFF SHAMPOO

Soapwort Shampoo (see page 81), combined with particular herbs, makes an excellent base for the treatment of this condition. Soapwort has a natural ability to cleanse itchy skin conditions such as dermatitis and dandruff.

Make an infusion from the following herbs and add the required amount, as directed in the recipe for the shampoo of your choice.

1 tablespoon dried peppermint
1 tablespoon dried parsley
2 tablespoons dried rosemary
2 tablespoons dried nettles
1 tablespoon dried thyme
2 litres (64 fl oz) boiling water

Essential oils will also help you get to the root of the problem. Rosemary or nutmeg oils massaged into the scalp are effective, and can be used in conjunction with the following shampoo:

30 ml (1 fl oz) olive oil
30 ml (1 fl oz) castor oil
180 ml (6 fl oz) rosemary infusion
6 drops rosemary oil
3 drops thyme oil
3 drops sage oil

Prepare the rosemary infusion, using 8 to 10 sprigs of fresh rosemary for 300 ml (10 fl oz) of boiling water. Add the required amount, as directed, to the Soapwort Shampoo, along with the oils and essential oils.

Both shampoos will help loosen the crusty layer of dead skin cells, which is then removed during the washing. They will also stimulate the healing mechanisms of the skin to help prevent a further buildup of dandruff.

AFTER-SHAMPOO CONDITIONING RINSE

Dandruff responds very well to treatment with herbal vinegar rinses.

Prepare the *Basic Recipe* for herbal vinegar (see Chapter One) with the following herbs:

equal quantities of rosemary, nettle, thyme, parsley
cider vinegar

Dilute the herbal vinegar 50:50 with distilled water and store in an airtight bottle.

After shampooing and thoroughly rinsing, massage a small quantity of the vinegar mixture well into your scalp. Between shampoos, massage about a teaspoon of this rinse into your scalp before going to bed.

AFTER-SHAMPOO ASTRINGENT RINSE

This astringent rinse is suitable for all hair types. It will close the pores and remove dandruff.

1 cup each of fresh comfrey, rosemary, sweet basil
125 ml (4 fl oz) cider vinegar
1 litre (32 fl oz) distilled water

Put the herbs and distilled water in an enamel or stainless steel saucepan, bring to the boil, cover and simmer for 15 minutes. Remove from the heat and allow to steep until cool. Strain through muslin, then drip through coffee filter paper and blend with the cider vinegar. Store in an airtight bottle.

After shampooing and rinsing, massage a small amount of the liquid well into your scalp.

ANTI-DANDRUFF CONDITIONING PASTE

For excessive flaking and irritating itching you may find the following paste helpful.

1 cup fresh nettle leaves, chopped
2 cups fresh rosemary leaves, finely minced
310 ml (10 fl oz) boiling water

Put the nettle leaves in a ceramic bowl, add the boiling water, cover and infuse until lukewarm. Add to a blender and liquidise. Return to the bowl and thoroughly mix in the rosemary with your fingers.

Massage the paste well into your scalp after shampooing. Leave in your hair for at least 10 minutes, then rinse out with the *Rosemary Hair Lotion* (see page 95).

SCALP OIL TREATMENT

This is a scalp conditioner so try to avoid spreading it through your hair.

30 ml (1 fl oz) castor oil
5 drops jojoba oil
5 drops carrot oil
5 drops evening primrose oil
5 drops rosemary oil

Warm the castor oil slightly and add the essential oils. Dip your fingers into the mixture and massage into your scalp every night before going to bed. Store the oil mixture in an amber-coloured glass bottle.

To warm the oil before use, stand the bottle in a container of hot water until it is sufficiently heated.

Setting Lotions

Herbal setting lotions set hair, especially if it has a natural tendency to be fine and limp. This recipe makes a gentle lotion for use on both dark and fair hair:

110 ml (3½ fl oz) Herb Water (see following)
5 ml (⅙ fl oz) glycerine
¼ teaspoon gum tragacanth
20 ml (⅔ fl oz) vodka

Add herb water to glycerine and stir until well blended. Dissolve the gum tragacanth in the vodka and then mix all liquids together. Store in a plastic pump-spray bottle and spray on dry hair before setting.

HERB WATER

DARK HAIR	FAIR HAIR
2 tablespoons fresh rosemary	*3 teaspoons dried chamomile*
625 ml (20 fl oz) distilled water	*625 ml (20 fl oz) distilled water*
3 drops rosemary oil	*1 tablespoon chopped lemon peel*

Put the rosemary or chamomile and distilled water in a stainless steel or enamel saucepan. Bring to the boil and simmer for 5 minutes. Remove from the heat and allow to steep until cool. Strain through muslin cloth and add rosemary oil or chopped lemon peel.

Oily Hair

Lemon juice is especially good for setting oily hair; far better than harsh hair sprays and lacquers. Squeeze and strain the juice of a lemon and comb through your hair before setting in rollers. Once the rollers have been removed, brush your hair and see how soft and silky it feels and looks.

SETTING LOTION FOR OILY HAIR

1 lemon
125 ml (4 fl oz) water
1 ml vodka

Cut the lemon into pieces and boil with the water in an enamel saucepan until reduced by half. Strain off the liquid and drip through filter paper. Add the vodka, which acts as a natural preservative. Store in a plastic pump-spray bottle.

Spray mist finely over your hair after styling. It dries quickly and will keep your hair in place.

To give your spray a delightful fragrance, add scented geranium oil, a drop at a time, until sufficiently scented.

DID YOU KNOW . . . ?

That shampoos and conditioning lotions containing rosemary extract will not only revitalise the scalp and hair but will also help to prevent dandruff.

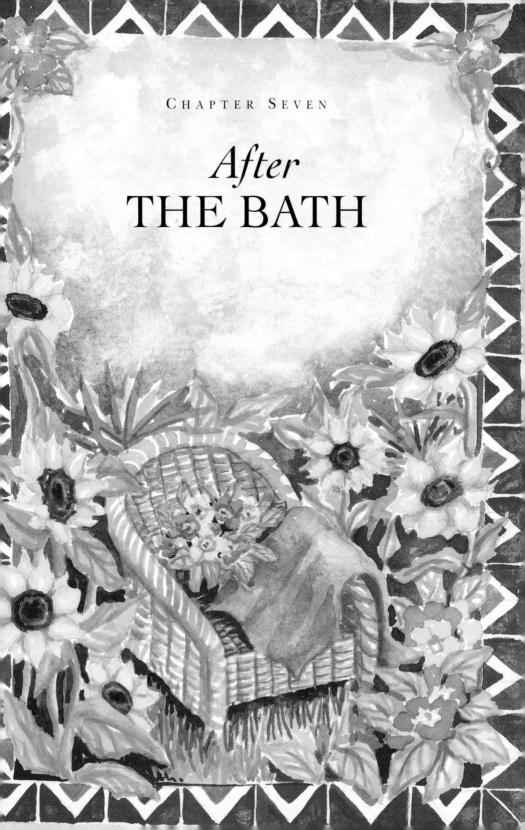

CHAPTER SEVEN

After
THE BATH

That Luxurious Feeling

Since the birth of cosmetic history human beings have pampered themselves after bathing with aromatic oils, lotions and powders.

Essential oils diluted in a vegetable oil leave the skin smelling wonderfully fragrant, and also give a golden gleam to the skin which no other substance, natural or synthetic, can reproduce. Choose essential oils to give you that perfect combination that will moisturise, nourish and soften your skin.

Body splashes and invigorating sprays or slap-on skin fresheners will lift your spirits on hot summer days and nights, or they can be used to simply tone your skin. The combination of essential oils, vinegar and water makes them particularly astringent and refreshing, and they can be formulated to suit whatever mood takes you.

After-bath body powders are a delight to use, and their mild deodorant properties and elusive scents will keep you feeling fresh and pampered. Using a natural deodorant will not prevent perspiration, but will control its unpleasant odour by inhibiting the growth of the micro-organisms which thrive on it.

To maintain that luxurious feeling of soft and smooth skin, use the following suggestions, or choose from any of the Body Oils in Chapter Four, or make your own special blends.

Body Oils

Make these by adding 1 drop of your chosen essential oil to every 1 ml of base vegetable oil. Ideal base oils to use are almond, apricot kernel and peach kernel, grapeseed, hazelnut, jojoba, olive, sesame, corn, soya and sunflower. Use cold-pressed oils for best results.

ALMOND OIL *Is the most popular base oil as it has little smell and is rich in protein. It is emollient, nourishing and slow to become rancid.*

APRICOT KERNEL *Has the same properties as almond oil, but is more expensive.*

PEACH KERNEL *Has the same properties as apricot kernel oil.*

GRAPESEED OIL *Is a very fine, clear oil that gives a satin-smooth finish without a greasy touch.*

HAZELNUT OIL *Penetrates the skin the most easily and deeply, stimulates the circulation and nourishes the skin.*

JOJOBA OIL	*Keeps well and gives a satin-smooth feel to the skin. It is more expensive than other oils.*
OLIVE OIL	*Is calming, warming, and good for rheumatism or for relieving itchy skin ailments. However, its scent may quite easily overpower the fragrance of the essential oils blended with it.*
SESAME OIL	*Keeps well, but its rich colour and odour may be off-putting.*
CORN, SOYA AND SUN-FLOWER OILS	*Cold-pressed corn oil is acceptable though rarely used. Soya has a nice feel and does not become sticky when massaged in. Sunflower oil has the least keeping qualities but does contain vitamin F. This vitamin controls your metabolic rate, takes care of your cholesterol balance, prevents eczema and regulates overactivity of the sebaceous glands.*

Other oils which can be added in small quantities to the base oil, apart from the essential oils, are:

AVOCADO OIL	*Is nourishing, penetrating and useful for fatty areas. It will become sticky if used in large quantities and massaged into a large area.*
CARROT OIL	*Is a natural tonic with rejuvenating qualities. Rich in many vitamins.*
EVENING PRIMROSE OIL	*Is useful for scaly skin.*
WHEATGERM OIL	*Is nourishing and rich in vitamin E, but is extremely oily on its own. Added in small quantities to your mixture it is a natural anti-oxidant (preservative) — 5 ml (1 teaspoon) added to every 50 ml (2 fl oz) of base oil will extend its keeping time.*

When making your own blends it is not necessary to add many different essential oils. Wonderful body oils can be achieved with just one aromatic oil, or a combination of up to five. Remember, the choice is yours, so let your nose, your mood and needs determine what will work best for you.

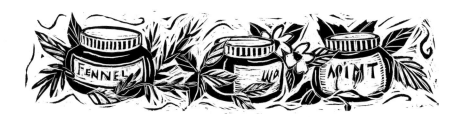

NORMAL SKIN

40 ml (1½ fl oz) almond oil
15 ml (½ fl oz) hazelnut oil
5 ml (⅙ fl oz) wheatgerm oil
20 drops rose oil
24 drops lavender
10 drops neroli
6 drops frankincense

OILY SKIN

40 ml (1½ fl oz) grapeseed oil
15 ml (½ fl oz) almond oil
5 ml (⅙ fl oz) wheatgerm oil
30 drops lemon oil
15 drops lavender oil
10 drops cypress oil
5 drops ylang-ylang oil

DRY SKIN

40 ml (1½ fl oz) almond oil
10 ml (⅓ fl oz) hazelnut oil
5 ml (⅙ fl oz) jojoba oil
5 ml (⅙ fl oz) wheatgerm oil
20 drops patchouli oil
20 drops rose oil
10 drops chamomile oil
10 drops carrot oil

BLEMISHED SKIN

40 ml (1½ fl oz) grapeseed oil
15 ml (½ fl oz) almond oil
5 ml (⅙ fl oz) wheatgerm oil
10 drops chamomile oil
10 drops lavender oil
15 drops geranium oil
15 drops calendula oil

TONING THE SKIN

Use this after-bath body oil to increase the elasticity of the skin and to promote the growth of new skin cells.

28 ml (1 fl oz) almond oil
2 ml (1/12 fl oz) wheatgerm oil
5 drops calendula oil
15 drops frankincense oil
5 drops lavender oil
5 drops chamomile oil

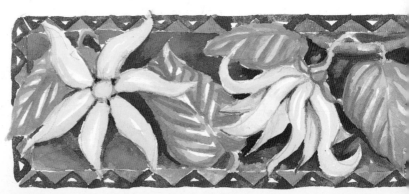

STRETCH MARKS

45 ml (1½ fl oz) almond oil
5 ml (⅙ fl oz) wheatgerm oil
5 drops neroli oil
10 drops frankincense oil
15 drops lavender oil

POST-DIET SAGGY SKIN

45 ml (1½ fl oz) almond oil
5 ml (⅙ fl oz) wheatgerm oil
5 drops carrot oil
9 drops lemongrass oil
8 drops pine oil
8 drops sage oil

MELANCHOLY

30 ml (1 fl oz) almond oil
5 drops chamomile oil
10 drops bergamot oil
5 drops neroli oil

Body Splashes

Floral vinegars diluted with distilled water and blended with aromatic oils
are extremely refreshing, ideal to splash on or spray liberally over your
skin. They leave your skin feeling soft, and they are highly effective as
deodorants and bactericides.

BASIC RECIPE

Prepare a floral or herbal vinegar (see Chapter One), using white wine
vinegar as the base. Choose from herbs such as basil, cloves, dill, scented
geranium leaves, honeysuckle flowers, jasmine flowers, lavender buds,
lemon verbena, rose petals, rosemary and violet.
  Dilute the vinegar in the following proportions:

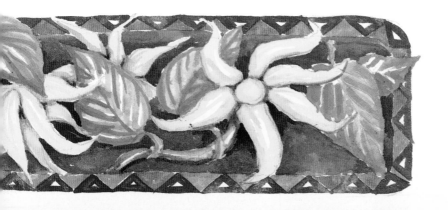

125 ml (4 fl oz) floral vinegar
10 ml (⅓ fl oz) vodka
625 ml (20 fl oz) distilled water
30 drops of selected essential oils

Store in a suitable airtight bottle or a plastic pump-spray bottle, and use on a fine mist setting.

Try one of the following body splashes, depending on your mood or needs.

SOOTHING

125 ml (4 fl oz) lavender vinegar (see Chapter One)
600 ml (20 fl oz) rose-water
10 ml (⅓ fl oz) vodka
10 drops lavender oil
10 drops rose oil
5 drops geranium oil
5 drops frankincense oil

Combine all ingredients in a glass bottle or jar, cap securely with a non-metallic lid, and shake thoroughly before use.

INVIGORATING

125 ml (4 fl oz) lemon verbena vinegar (see Chapter One)
625 ml (20 fl oz) distilled water
10 ml (⅓ fl oz) vodka
10 drops lime oil
10 drops lavender oil
5 drops lemon oil
5 drops lemongrass oil

Prepare as for *Soothing Body Splash.*

SUMMER SPECIAL

This delightful fruity splash is refreshing and uplifting, ideal to use on those hot and sticky summer days, after showering, or when you have been at the beach.

125 ml (4 fl oz) rose vinegar (see page 6)
600 ml (20 fl oz) orange flower water (see page 6)
10 ml (⅓ fl oz) vodka

10 drops orange oil
10 drops mandarin oil
5 drops lemon oil
5 drops grapefruit oil

Prepare as for *Soothing Body Splash.*

Body Powders

Body powders first became fashionable in Elizabethan times, when they were not only used to scent the body but were also rubbed liberally on clothes and gloves. Make your own aromatic powders, and enjoy the feeling of your skin being luxuriously pampered.

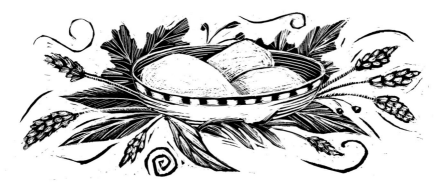

FRAGRANT DUSTING POWDER
75 g (2½ oz) rice flour
75 g (2½ oz) cornflour
1 tablespoon powdered orrisroot
5 ml (⅙ fl oz) essential oil of choice
3 teaspoons lovage water (see Herbal Infusions, *page 3)*

Mix the dry ingredients. Add the essential oil and lovage water and mix them through until the powder feels dry. Extra oil can be added if the scent is not strong enough, but take care not to get the mixture too wet. If it does become a little too wet, adjust by adding more dry ingredients, a little at a time. Once dry, sieve twice, store in a box and apply with a large dusting puff.

ROSE AFTER-BATH POWDER
90 g (3 oz) French chalk
50 g (2 oz) cornflour
4 g magnesium carbonate
6 g calcium carbonate
1 tablespoon powdered orrisroot
15 ml (½ fl oz) lovage water
5 ml (⅙ fl oz) rose oil

Prepare as for the *Fragrant Dusting Powder*. Store in a plastic bottle with holes punched in the lid.

Note: Magnesium carbonate and calcium carbonate are both available from the chemist.

Herbal Deodorant

An effective deodorant can be made by steeping herbs in cider vinegar, (see *Herb and Flower Vinegars*, Chapter One). This will have both a subdued perfume and antiseptic properties, thus helping you feel fresh and odour-free.

Herbs suitable for making deodorant vinegars are rosemary and thyme combined, lavender, sage, lovage, eau de Cologne mint, spearmint, scented geranium leaves, eucalyptus, marjoram and honeysuckle.

LIQUID DEODORANT
10 ml (⅓ fl oz) herb vinegar (see page 6)
80 ml (2½ fl oz) distilled water

Store in a tightly sealed bottle.

After washing and drying underarms, dab on the vinegar and allow to dry.

DID YOU KNOW . . . ?
That a natural deodorant controls odour by inhibiting the growth of micro-organisms which thrive on the skin, but still allows the body to perspire naturally?

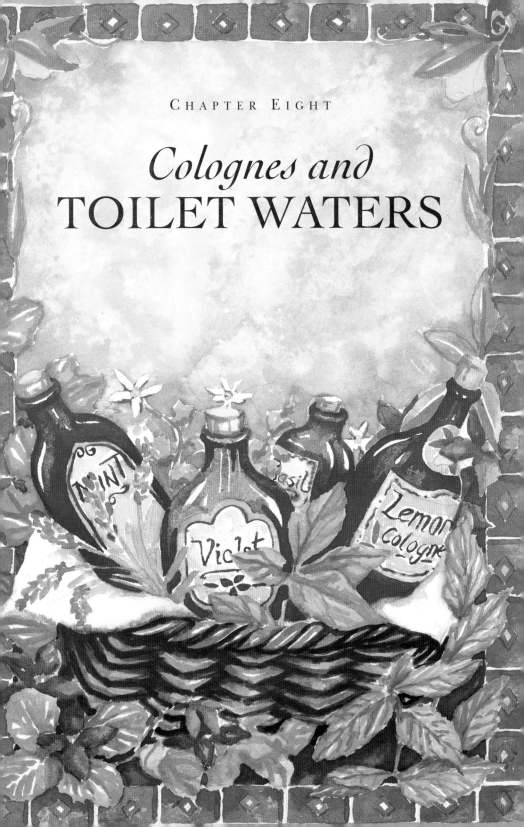

CHAPTER EIGHT

Colognes and TOILET WATERS

Scents to Refresh and Enjoy

Flowers and herbs can be made into colognes and perfumes that are a delight to use. When splashed onto your body after a wash or bath their refreshing fragrance will lift your spirits, and make you feel special.

Perfumes have been used throughout history to mask body odours and to increase attractiveness. They were made by distilling, by steeping herbs and flowers, or by mixing aromatic oils with alcohol. One of the simplest ways to make your own toilet water or cologne is to add essential oils to alcohol or to a mixture of alcohol and distilled water.

It is illegal to purchase or to distil pure alcohol. However, you can make an acceptable perfume using a high proof vodka. Experiment first by adding essential oils of your choice, drop by drop, to plain water until you find a scent that is acceptable to you.

Remember, though, blending essential oils is an art on its own and the best perfumers in the world take their work as seriously as any great painter or other artist. The careful mixture of base, middle and top notes is a symphony of aromatic elements, with subtle undertones and lingering highlights that come together to tantalise and please. You cannot master the perfumer's art from the limited information in this text but, with patience, you too will be able to develop your own exciting fragrances.

Your first experiments in mixing essential oils should be limited to no more than three or four scents at a time. Make sure you test them on parts of your skin that are as far away from each other as possible so the scents do not blend with one another and confuse your nose. Choose scents that match your mood and that are appropriate for the time of day. I suggest refreshing scents, such as the citrus oils, or even the delicate floral notes like rose, are best used in the morning. The heavier oriental or spice scents such as musk and patchouli are best in the evening.

It is the harmonious blending of the different notes that makes a good perfume. Top notes evaporate fast, middle notes not so fast, and base notes slowly. So it is important when making a perfume to first establish your base note, or a combination of base notes, followed by your middle and top.

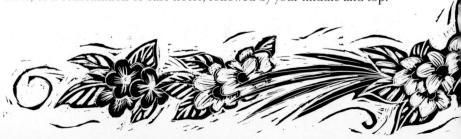

Here is a list of some essential oils which you may like to experiment with, and their appropriate categories:

BASE NOTES	MIDDLE NOTES	TOP NOTES
Cedarwood	Chamomile	Thyme
Cinnamon	Cypress	Basil
Frankincense	Geranium	Bergamot
Patchouli	Hyssop	Mandarin
Benzoin	Carnation	Sage
Camphor	Clary Sage	Peppermint
Clove	Rosemary	Niaouli
Ginger	Pine	Neroli
Jasmine	Melissa	Amoise
Myrrh	Lemongrass	Chamomile (Roman)
Rose	Linden	Lemon
Sandalwood	Nutmeg	Coriander
Ylang-Ylang	Lavender	Lavender
	Sweet Marjoram	Lime
	Juniper	Spearmint
	Violet	

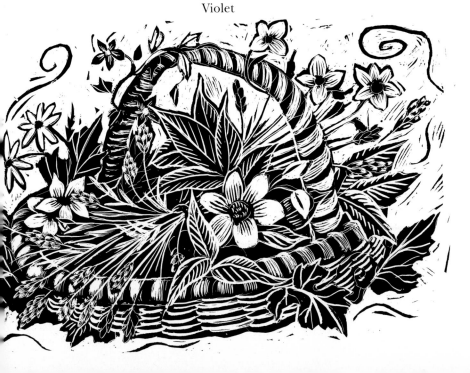

A Little Guidance

When blending essential oils, a general rule of thumb would be a ratio of 4 parts top note, 2 parts middle note and 1 part base note. If the scent is too fresh, add a little base note. If it is too heavy, add a little middle or top note. Go slowly, sparingly and use very small amounts always.

Remember to write down what you do — you may create a masterpiece!

Making Colognes and Toilet Waters

If the prospect of blending your own perfumes is too daunting, try the following recipes. Use them as they are or experiment with them to suit your personal taste.

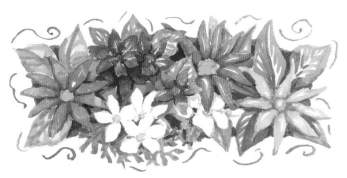

FLORAL TOILET WATER

This is a delightful, simple-to-make toilet water, that uses either fresh or dried flowers of your choice.

1 litre (32 fl oz) distilled water
flower petals, sufficient
40 ml (1½ fl oz) vodka

Boil the distilled water in an enamel or stainless steel saucepan. Fill a warmed, heatproof jar with the flower petals, then add the distilled water. Seal and leave to cool slightly. Add the vodka, seal again and leave until completely cold. Strain through muslin and then drip through coffee filter paper.

Store in a suitable attractive glass bottle. The old-fashioned ones with ground glass stoppers are ideal.

CARMELITE WATER

This is an old-fashioned recipe based on the one invented by the Carmelite monks in Paris in 1611.

1 generous handful angelica leaves
1 generous handful lemon balm leaves
15 g (½ oz) bruised coriander seeds
1 nutmeg, minced
2 tablespoons cloves
3 pieces of cinnamon stick, crushed
310 ml (10 fl oz) high proof vodka
155 ml (5 fl oz) distilled water

Put all the herbs and spices in a wide-mouthed glass jar, add the vodka, seal, and shake vigorously. Leave in a warm place for one week to 10 days, shaking every day. Strain through muslin, then drip through coffee filter paper and dilute with the distilled water.

Store in an attractive glass bottle.

ROSE AND LAVENDER COLOGNE

1 litre (32 fl oz) vodka
10 drops clove oil
15 drops lavender oil
15 drops rose oil
500 ml (16 fl oz) distilled water

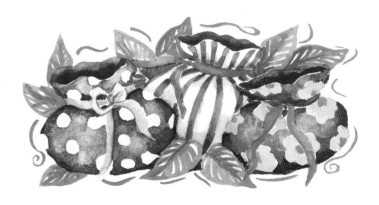

Put the vodka in a suitable bottle, add the essential oils, seal, then shake vigorously and allow to stand for one week. Add the distilled water, seal, shake again and leave for a further two weeks. Drip through coffee filter paper.

INVIGORATING LEMON COLOGNE

This is a refreshing, cooling skin cologne to use after your shower on hot summer days, or to splash on simply to lift your spirits.

500 ml (16 fl oz) distilled water
2 cups fresh (tightly packed) lemon balm
1 litre (32 fl oz) vodka
20 drops lemon oil
10 drops lime oil

Prepare a herbal infusion with the lemon balm and distilled water (see Chapter One).

Put the vodka in a suitable bottle, add the essential oils, seal and leave to stand for one week. Add the herbal infusion, reseal, shake vigorously and leave to stand for a further two weeks. Drip through coffee filter paper.

LAVENDER TOILET WATER

500 ml (16 fl oz) distilled water
50 g (2 oz) dried lavender buds
310 ml (10 fl oz) vodka
6 drops lavender oil

Prepare a herbal infusion (see Chapter One) with the lavender buds and distilled water. Mix the lavender infusion and vodka together in a suitable bottle, add the lavender oil, seal and leave to stand for two weeks. Drip through coffee filter paper and rebottle.

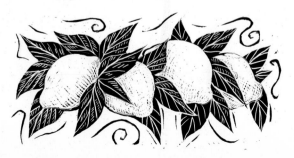

SPRING FLOWERS SKIN FRESHENER

2 cups of fresh violet petals, or 1 cup dried
1 cup fresh rose petals, or ½ cup dried
25 g (1 oz) cassia bark
375 ml (12 fl oz) vodka
14 drops violet oil
14 drops bergamot oil
750 ml (24 fl oz) distilled water

Put the flower petals and cassia bark in a wide-mouthed glass jar and add the vodka. Seal, and leave in a warm place for one week. Strain, squeezing all the alcohol from petals, and rebottle. Add the essential oils and distilled water, seal and allow to stand for another week. Drip through coffee filter paper.

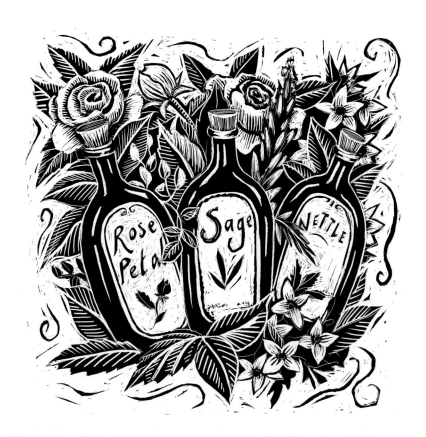

Glossary

AROMATIC	*Having an agreeable fragrant odour.*
ASTRINGENT	*Contracting organic tissue, reducing secretions and discharges.*
BENZOIN TINCTURE	*Has preservative properties; is also a powerful astringent and has the effect of emulsifying wool fat (lanolin).*
CARRIER OIL	*Base oil to which a quantity of essential oil has been added.*
DECOCTION	*Extract of substance obtained by boiling.*
DISTILLATION	*Extraction of pure essence of a herb or flower obtained by evaporation and condensation.*
EMOLLIENT	*Substance used externally to soften and soothe.*
EMULSIFY	*To finely disperse oil, and then combine it completely with another solution.*
EMULSION	*Fine dispersion of one liquid in another.*
ESSENCE	*Extract obtained by distillation.*
ESSENTIAL OIL	*Volatile oil found in herbs, giving them their characteristic aroma.*
EXFOLIATE	*Remove layers of dead skin cells.*
FLOWER WATER	*A fragrant herb or flower water made by distillation, infusion or decoction.*
FULLER'S EARTH	*Has binding properties; is used in natural cosmetics for its astringent and stimulating effect on the skin.*
INFUSION	*Diluted liquid extract from the steeping of a herb or flower in boiling water.*
LOTION	*Liquid preparation used externally.*
SEBACEOUS GLAND	*Skin duct conveying oily matter to lubricate skin and hair.*
SEBUM	*Secretion of sebaceous glands.*
TONIC	*Substance or mixture which has an overall beneficial or invigorating effect on the body.*
VOLATILE OIL	*Essence obtained from herbs and flowers.*

Index of Recipes

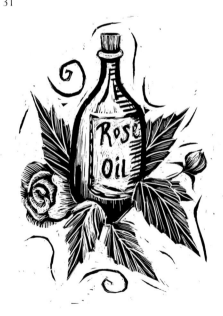

About the author

Alan Hayes' interest in herbs first began as a teenager, when he became aware, through his grandmother, of the herbal lore that had been passed down through the Hayes family for generations. Alan's interest grew as he studied herbal medicines and natural therapies, and his expertise expanded. On this basis, he has now established a reasonably self-sufficient lifestyle for himself and his family.

Using the knowledge gained from his study and from family records, Alan has become the successful author of a number of books on herbal lore and healing, notably the bestseller *It's So Natural*, an A to Z compilation of environmentally-friendly hints, tips and remedies for the home, health and garden, based on the author's widely syndicated and popular weekly column of the same name. More recently, Alan has published *Country Scents* which brings the magic and colour of herbs into the home and garden, in an easy-to-read, step-by-step format that allows the reader to capture the charms of yesteryear with natural products.

With an ever growing number of people interested in natural health care, Alan has continued to write on this subject, so that others may benefit from his knowledge and experience in this fascinating area.